HORMONE HEALTH FOR ALL AGES

DISCOVER HOW TO NATURALLY BALANCE YOUR HORMONES THROUGH DIET AND LIFESTYLE FOR AUTOIMMUNE AND OTHER HEALTH DEFICIENCIES

ELIZABETH HERZOG

Copyright © 2023 by Elizabeth Herzog

All rights reserved. No portion of this book may be reproduced in any form without permission from the publisher, except as permitted by US copyright law. For permissions contact lizzy4252@yahoo.com

Published by Elizabeth Herzog in the United States of America.

This book is intended purely for educational and entertainment purposes. The information in this book is not intended as a substitute for medical advice. It is not intended to diagnose or treat injuries or medical conditions, nor is the information intended to replace advice and treatments from a licensed healthcare professional. Readers should consult the advice of a licensed healthcare professional for injury, illness, and other health conditions. The author and publisher assume no direct or indirect responsibility or liability for any consequences of using the information or advice in this book.

TABLE OF CONTENTS

Author's Note	5
Introduction	7

1. LET'S TALK ABOUT HORMONES! — 15
Your endocrine system made simple	16
Hormone imbalance is annoying . . . and worse!	24
Snapshots of your hormones through your life	28

2. THE ESTROGEN MYTH — 33
Enter progestin	34
Introducing HRT	36
Sara's story	47

3. THE ANSWER: NATURAL PROGESTERONE — 53
Progesterone's role in your body	54
Progesterone and your bones	56
What causes unbalanced progesterone?	58
Signs you may have low progesterone	60
Can you replace progesterone with synthetic progestin?	65
Josie's story	66
Boost your natural progesterone	70

4. ESTROGEN DOMINANCE — 73
How estrogen took over the world	74
Signs and symptoms of estrogen dominance	77
Daniel's story	80
Xenoestrogens are changing our wildlife	83
An unprecedented problem in human history	85

5. HORMONES & AUTOIMMUNE DISEASE 89
   Hormones and your immune system 92
   Genetics and autoimmune issues 99
   My road to hell and back 101

6. HORMONE BALANCE MADE SIMPLE 109
   Diet 111
   Stress 127
   Exercise 135
   Sleep 138
   Environmental toxins 141
   Daily schedule for hormone balance 150
   Your path to healing 153

Afterword 155
About the Author 157
References 159

AUTHOR'S NOTE

This book is about a topic that's often misunderstood and considered taboo: women's hormone health—from periods to fertility, orgasm, menopause, and beyond. The official sources I've found on these topics are usually laughably misinformed.

That's one reason I decided to write this book.

For over 25 years, I worked in and owned several natural health stores. Customers often came to me with questions they couldn't ask anyone else. Maybe their doctors had told them their symptoms weren't real, weren't a problem, or would go away naturally. Sometimes my customer was too uncomfortable to even talk to her doctor. Either way, I was "safe" for her: I was nonjudgmental and willing to help her on a one-on-one basis.

Most of my customers were women going through

menopause, struggling with fertility, or suffering through irregular periods. Many had low libidos and couldn't reach orgasm. Their problems were so similar that I started hosting PowerPoint presentations over lunch to explain common problems and solutions. These lunches were popular! I quickly realized that women of all ages were desperate to talk to each other. They wanted to share what they knew and what confused them about their own bodies. The space I created was a modern-day version of women's circles that have existed throughout history.

Writing this book is a way to expand that circle, sharing knowledge that can help all women everywhere (and the men and children they love). I've filled it with many years worth of knowledge I built up while running vitamin shops, and through earning my certification in functional nutrition. I'm not a doctor and I'm thankful for that. Doctors are important, and I would never suggest foregoing medical treatment when necessary. But as you'll learn in the stories ahead, natural healers have knowledge that doctors simply don't.

I hope this book answers your questions and sets you on a journey to healing!

INTRODUCTION

"Great spirits have always encountered opposition from mediocre minds."

— ALBERT EINSTEIN

In 2000, I was running a popular natural health shop in Fresno, California. We sold vitamins, herbs, and supplements, and our staff was well educated in every product on our shelves. We were the local go-to source for not only natural health products, but also for reliable, safe, educated advice—especially for people who couldn't find answers with traditional Western medicine.

One day, a woman approached me as I stocked progesterone cream in the women's health aisle. She looked to be in her late forties or early fifties. "Are you Liz?" she asked, a friendly but troubled look in her clear blue eyes.

"You found me!" I said, giving her my full attention.

"My name's Sally. My friend told me you're the one to talk to about hormone problem?"

I reassured her that she was in the right place. I had helped hundreds of women of all ages balance their hormones:

- Young women who weren't having periods.
- Women who couldn't get pregnant.
- New mothers struggling with postpartum depression and low libido.
- Women with excessive bleeding and anemia.
- Women going through menopause.
- Postmenopausal women.
- I'd even helped men and children with hormone-related issues!
- I'd seen it *all!*

A glimmer of hope crept into Sally's eyes, but she wasn't quite confident yet. I could tell she had been through the wringer and doubted that anyone could help her.

"Oh, good," she said. "I've been struggling with my hormones for a few years now. Lately, it's gotten worse. I'm at my wit's end."

Knowing how women in Sally's shoes were often ignored

or brushed aside by their doctors, I encouraged her to open up. "Well, we can't have you stuck at your wit's end! Tell me what's up."

What she said next didn't surprise me.

"I've been gaining weight, even though I'm eating healthy, and my exercise routine hasn't changed. My emotions are all over the place. The other day I got so mad at my husband that I threw a bread roll at him! He forgave me and we laughed it off. But later I felt so sad I was practically in tears. And Liz . . . *I never want to have sex anymore.* I still love him, but it's like my libido has just disappeared. When we do have sex, it almost feels like a chore. I know he can sense I'm not into it, and I'm so worried that it's going to create distance between us, or that he'll go somewhere else—maybe to someone younger—to get what I'm not giving. Do you think this is happening because I'm doing something wrong? Maybe I drank too much in college and it's catching up with me? Or just because I'm aging?"

"Definitely not!" I said. "It's not your fault, and none of what you've described has to come with healthy aging. Have you talked to your doctor about this?"

"Yes, but he says there's nothing wrong! He said my blood work is 'normal,' and he just wanted to put me on HRT for more estrogen."

"That doesn't surprise me," I said, suppressing an eye roll.

"I trust science," Sally said, "but I'm just not sure about HRT. I don't want to load my body up with harsh pharmaceuticals. Do you think I'm being . . . high maintenance? Or irrational?"

"Okay, let's get *that* out of your head right now," I said. "Wanting to be responsible about your health is *not* high maintenance or irrational."

She let out a big sigh of relief. "Thank you! I don't want to just slap a band-aid on the symptoms. I want to get to the root of what's going on."

"We can do that," I said. I could practically see the weight drop off her shoulders.

Does any part of Sally's story sound familiar? It was one of thousands I heard while running my natural health businesses—a path I started walking over 25 years ago.

My journey began when my father bought a health food store and asked me to help run it. I couldn't say yes fast enough! Getting to spend all day around herbs and supplements? Becoming an expert on the body and its relationship to the mind, heart, and Mother Nature? Yes, please! I already loved all things natural health, but I could never have guessed how much the store would change my life. The new job gave me permission to indulge my passion, and I soaked up *all* the knowledge I could. Before I knew it, people were coming to me for advice . . . and I actually knew what to tell them! Better yet, customers would often come back to thank me, saying their issues had cleared up.

I learned what millennia of healers have experienced through the ages: helping people is one of the most fulfilling purposes a person can have. I decided to study alternative medicine more seriously, and in two years, I was a certified naturopath. That meant I could teach others! (There's a difference between certified and licensed naturopaths. My certification means I can teach twenty-five classes a week if I want. But I don't have a license to treat patients.)

I taught classes on all kinds of health topics right there in my store. But my most popular classes by far were about women's hormone health. No surprise there! I had already talked to a lot of women, and I knew that so many of our health issues come down to one thing: hormone imbalances.

Word of mouth is my favorite form of advertising. Soon, the women I had helped were telling their friends about me. It wasn't long until I was the go-to source for hormone health, helping women every day. There was Kathy, who I helped move through menopause gracefully. (Did you know that hot flashes are unheard of in some countries? I'll tell you the secret in Chapter 3!)

There was Josie, a woman in her late teens who had stopped having periods but was about to get married and wanted to have children. Using information you'll find in this book, we were able to get her periods started and get her pregnant. She's now a happy mother of five.

Then there was Sara, a new mother struggling to pull herself out of postpartum depression. By shifting her to a new lifestyle and supplement routine (and sticking with the routine over several months), we managed to balance her hormones and help her fall in love with her baby . . . and with life!

You'll find more stories throughout the book. Most of the women's names are changed, but their stories represent the most common problems I saw while working in three consecutive natural health stores. These women's smiles blend together for me in a beautiful tapestry of memory. It broke my heart that the Western medical system had failed them so utterly. Although the good people in that system may have tried their best, they simply didn't have the knowledge or tools to help.

I'll never forget when I went to visit a doctor for a consultation to have my tubes tied. Before my appointment, the doctor called me into his office and sat me down at his desk. I'll admit, I was a little nervous. But this doctor was young and pretty good-looking, so that helped!

"You're Liz Herzog?" he asked.

"Yes," I said.

"The Liz Herzog who works at B-Alive Vitamins?"

I was surprised that he knew my store! "Yes . . . am I in trouble?"

He laughed, showing a perfect row of sparkly white teeth. "Not at all! I wanted to meet you! So many of my patients tell me they talked to you and that you helped them. The way their issues are clearing up is amazing. So I have to ask you . . . what are you giving them?"

What a relief! Not only was I not in trouble—I was also being asked for advice! Then followed a friendly heart-to-heart about women's health, hormones, and all the information and supplements I wish more Western doctors showed an interest in. I was filling a very real and very big need in my community. Considering all the advancements we've made in the fields of science and medicine, this gap in knowledge is disappointing. There are good doctors (like the attractive guy I went to, ooh-la-la!), but on the whole, Western medicine has let women down.

I've poured over 20 years of knowledge into this book. Whatever your age, wherever you are in your hormone health journey, the information here can help you. This is the wisdom that millennia of women have understood and passed down to their daughters and granddaughters. We lost touch with it when men were put in charge of women's medicine (they do their best, the poor dears). And we *really* got off track when Western medicine started trying to solve problems without understanding how women's hormones work in the first place.

What are their solutions to problems they don't understand? HRT (hormone replacement therapy), birth control pills, a never-ending parade of pharmaceutical drugs, and way too many hysterectomies. It's insane! Our ancestral foremothers are rolling in their graves!

This book is your ticket back to sanity.

In these pages, you'll learn:

- Supplements to help balance hormone-related issues.
- The #1 PRODUCT I put almost everyone on.

- Common hormone myths that even doctors get wrong.
- Home products to toss in the trash today to stop disrupting hormones.
- What to eat to balance your hormones.
- How to have the best sex of your life (and why it's important for your hormones).
- And a lot more!

The relationship you have with your body is the most important one in your life. Your body is a super-responsive, intuitive animal, *and it's on your side.*

This book is written in a clear, accessible, easy-to-use style. After you finish reading (and put the advice into practice!), you'll understand your body more clearly than you ever have in the past. You'll know what natural products and routines will best support it. You'll even be able to help the men and children in your life who struggle with hormone issues.

Most of all, *you'll feel like yourself again*—and the best version of yourself, too. The healthy, vibrant, emotionally open, and sexy woman you know you are. When your hormones are imbalanced, it can profoundly affect every aspect of your life. And when you bring them back into balance, every area of your life flourishes in response.

Here's to your health and happiness!

1

LET'S TALK ABOUT HORMONES!

"The doctor of the future will give no medicine, but will instruct his patients in care of the human frame, in diet, and in the cause and prevention of disease."

— THOMAS EDISON

Did you know that hormones affect way more than just your reproductive health?

Hormones affect (let me take a deep breath before sharing this list!): skin health, hair growth, blood pressure, blood sugar, bone health, metabolism, weight and fat distribution, appetite, sleep, stress levels, mood, mental focus, muscle mass, and more. And that's in addition to reproductive-related stuff like fertility, vaginal dryness, the menstrual cycle, sex drive, orgasm, puberty, and menopause.

If even one or two of the issues I just mentioned are out of whack, it can affect your entire life. If you can't sleep so you're late for work, your boss isn't going to be too happy with you! If you're constantly moody and not interested in sex, your partner is going to wonder what's up . . . and maybe spend a few nights in the guest room to "give you some space." If your hair gets thin and starts breaking, that's going to affect your self-image.

Hormones have an all-encompassing impact on our lives.

I found that most of the women coming into my natural health stores for advice had problems that stemmed from hormone issues. Women asking me about facial hair, joint pain, or weight gain were sometimes surprised when I gave them the same product that I recommended for women trying to regulate their periods or stop hot flashes. It often comes down to healthy, happy hormones.

YOUR ENDOCRINE SYSTEM MADE SIMPLE

Don't worry—I'm not going to get too sciencey on you! But before we get into all the ways your hormones affect your body throughout your life, I want to lay a little groundwork, so you understand what these hormones are, their different functions, and how your body produces them. You can always come back and review this information again.

A simple explanation of your endocrine system is that it's made up of glands that produce hormones. Here's a beginner-friendly overview of what they do for you[1]:

- **Pituitary** – The head honcho in charge of monitoring your hormone levels. If something gets out of balance, your pituitary sends out orders to "get back in line!" Your pituitary gland is no bigger than a pea and is located beneath your brain.
- **Hypothalamus** – If your pituitary gland is the king of hormone balance, think of the hypothalamus as the "power behind the throne." It keeps pituitary hormones regulated. It also plays a role in blood pressure, sleep, appetite, fluid retention, and more. It's located at the base of your brain just above your pituitary.
- **Ovaries** – Release the sex hormones estrogen and progesterone, influencing fertility, your period, mood, breast growth, fat distribution (they give women a curvy shape), sex drive, and all things feminine health. You have one on each side of your uterus.
- **Testes** – Produce testosterone to influence all things masculine health, including sex drive, stress, muscle growth, hair growth, weight, and more. The testes are in an external pouch (the scrotum) to regulate their temperature and keep sperm healthy.

- **Thyroid and parathyroid** – These two are responsible for your metabolism and calcium levels, producing thyroid hormones and PTH (peptide hormones). They're in the front of your neck and below your larynx.
- **Adrenal** – Creates stress hormones (like cortisol) so you can fight or flee from danger, keeps your energy levels balanced (so you don't feel fatigued all the time), and affects metabolism and blood pressure. There's one adrenal gland on top of each of your kidneys.
- **Pineal body** – Makes melatonin to regulate your sleep cycles. It's in the middle of your brain below your corpus callosum.
- **Pancreas** – Regulates your blood sugar by producing insulin (which is a hormone). It also plays a role in digestion. Your pancreas is behind your stomach.

Your organs can produce hormones, too—including your stomach, intestines, kidneys, and heart. It's not their main job, but that doesn't mean they have no impact. Even fat produces hormones!

You can see that your endocrine system isn't like your vascular system, with isolated pathways through the body. It's a holistic system integrated throughout your entire body. It cannot be considered separately. Your endocrine system is constantly working to keep all of your physiological processes balanced. The tools the endocrine system uses to accomplish this never-ending task are hormones.

Think of hormones as little messengers. A hormone contains information. It travels through your bloodstream to its destination (hormones have their own internal GPS systems, they always know where to go!), and locks into a receptor cell on an organ. Then the hormone shares its information and tells the organ what to do.

Your sex hormones

Three main sex hormones influence your reproductive health. From puberty through menopause and beyond, these "three amigas" are running the show. You've probably heard of them!

They are:

- Estrogen
- Progesterone
- Testosterone

Estrogen

Estrogen is responsible for your secondary sex characteristics, including the development of your breasts, and weight distribution around your hips and thighs (giving you curves). It helps keep your periods regular and grows the lining of your uterus nice and thick so a fertilized egg can implant. It keeps your vaginal walls thick and lubricated, so sex feels good. It also affects your cholesterol, blood sugar, bone and muscle mass, collagen, mental focus, and more.

Most estrogen is produced in your ovaries.

There are actually three types of estrogen[2]:

- **Estradiol** – The main type of estrogen your body makes during your reproductive years (it's very potent!).
- **Estriol** – This type is prevalent when you get pregnant.
- **Estrone** – Your body makes this type after menopause.

While doctors understand a lot about estrogen, I want *you* to understand that some of their information is . . . well . . . less than reliable.

There's a prevailing belief among medical minds (I'll be polite and refrain from calling them "med heads!") that low estrogen is a major problem for women, especially as we age. This is just plain not true. In most cases, our bodies are struggling to metabolize *too much* estrogen, including the estrogen our bodies produce and all the xenoestrogens in our environment (these are chemicals your body treats like estrogen—more on them later!). This misunderstanding leads to a lot of bad advice. For example, many medical professionals believe that low estrogen leads to osteoporosis, so you should take estrogen to protect your bones as you age. This is not how the body works. The idea that estrogen protects against bone loss means doctors are prescribing HRT left and right... but HRT doesn't solve the problem.

The real bone-building hormone is progesterone.

Progesterone

Ask your doctor about progesterone, and she'll probably tell you some of the most popularly known information about it: After you ovulate, your ovaries create progesterone. Its job is to regulate your periods and make sure your body is the perfect environment for a fertilized egg. If you get pregnant, progesterone's job description gets bigger. It supports the endometrium and the placenta (which also starts pumping out progesterone), stops you from getting pregnant when you're already pregnant, and tells your body it's time to start lactating.

What your doctor may not mention (or even be aware of) is that progesterone has a much bigger influence on your overall health. She's thinking of progesterone like the lead violinist in an orchestra... when it's really more like the conductor! It plays a role in libido, cancer prevention (especially uterine cancer), reducing fibrocystic breasts and uterine fibroids, skin and hair health, blood clotting, fat burning, mood, bone health, having a healthy, graceful, low-stress menopause, and more.

As we'll discuss later in this book, progesterone is the great balancer of estrogen. Most women I've spoken to are dealing with high estrogen and low progesterone.

Testosterone

Yup, you need testosterone, too! Women don't have anywhere near as much of this hormone as men, but a little goes a long way. It's made in our ovaries and adrenal glands, and it supports libido, muscle and bone health, mood, concentration, and energy levels. It's one of several male hormones classified as androgens.

Endocrine disorders

Considering all the glands and hormones that are constantly interacting, your endocrine system does a remarkable job of keeping your body and mind balanced. It's like a big team of acrobats all working together to flip each other through the air! But the balance is delicate. If even one acrobat falls or shows up late to his mark, the whole team can crash into the ground.

Here are a few endocrine disorders you may have heard of[3]:

- **PCOS** – Polycystic ovarian syndrome. If your body produces too many androgens (male hormones), a lot of tiny cysts grow on your ovaries. You may ovulate irregularly or not at all. It leads to pain, acne, weight gain, hair growth (some women with PCOS shave their faces), and in some cases, infertility and diabetes.[3]
- **Diabetes** – When your pancreas doesn't make enough insulin (or your body doesn't respond to

your insulin very well), you can't easily process the sugar in your bloodstream.[3]
- **Osteoporosis** – Your bones are losing density and growing brittle. As I mentioned earlier, most doctors believe osteoporosis is caused by low estrogen as women age. The real cause is low progesterone.[3]
- **Low testosterone** – You won't usually hear this called by its official name, and for good reason. "Hypogonadism" is a mouthful! It develops when the testes don't create enough testosterone. This affects a man's sex drive (and his ability to get an erection), muscle strength, and mental capacity.[3]
- **Thyroid disorders** – If your thyroid is producing too many or too few hormones, you'll get hyperthyroidism (too many) or hypothyroidism (not enough). Both conditions affect your weight, energy levels, and heart health. Some people with thyroid disorders develop goiters.[3]

I also want to mention endocrine disruptors, aka "xenoestrogens." We'll talk more about these in Chapter 4, but they deserve a quick mention here. Endocrine disruptors are man-made chemicals that mess with your hormones: increasing them, decreasing them, blocking them altogether, mimicking them, or changing the way they're produced.

Endocrine disruptors show up practically everywhere.

Our society is using these chemicals in everything because they're cheap, convenient, and make products last longer. A walk through your typical grocery store or Target is a tour of endocrine disruptors. They're in house cleaners, pesticides, food packaging, the food itself, cosmetics, shampoo, perfume, plastics, carpets, clothing, and even in our water and air.

Repeat after me: *Hormone issues are not your fault.* A woman's body is a delicate balance of holistic processes. It's tough to maintain that balance even without being exposed to a minefield of endocrine disrupters every day!

HORMONE IMBALANCE IS ANNOYING . . . AND WORSE!

Let's talk about a few ways that hormone imbalances can affect your life.

Cell regeneration

HGH (Human Growth Hormone) is made in the pituitary gland. Both men and women have it. I'll bet you can guess what it's in charge of . . . Your growth and cellular regeneration!

HGH is most active in children, helping them grow a lot of cells and shoot up like little bean sprouts. For adults, it affects everything from your metabolism to your muscles, to your skin, bones, and more. A lot of athletes want to take HGH since it helps build muscle and keeps them feeling young and strong. For women, it also helps regulate estrogen and progesterone.

But as women age, our pituitary glands make less HGH. That means it's not telling your body to regrow your cells as quickly. Low levels of HGH can lead to weight gain, reduced muscle mass, low bone density, thin and sagging skin, and more.

Sexual function

Never in the mood to get frisky? It's your hormones! Is your vagina too dry to have sex comfortably? You can get high-quality lube to fill in, but don't ignore the sign that your hormones are imbalanced. Can't come as easily as you used to? Again, blame your hormones.

Hormone imbalance—especially estrogen dominance— can lead to low libido, vaginal dryness, and even the inability to orgasm. Talk about frustrating! It can seriously affect your relationship, your pleasure, and your self-image.

Reproduction

A lot of hormones are involved in pregnancy. If any one of them steps out of line the entire production can grind to a halt.

Too much estrogen can interfere with ovulation or prevent it altogether (that's called anovulation). If you're not ovulating, your eggs aren't being released from your ovaries. Hormone imbalances can also make your eggs slow to mature (or prevent maturation altogether), lead to a thin uterine lining that isn't a healthy environment for a fertilized egg, and cause abnormal bleeding, spotting, and even miscarriage.

Thyroid issues can disrupt your menstrual cycle, and

high levels of prolactin (the breast milk-stimulating hormone) can stop you from ovulating naturally.

Mood and mental health

How many times have we as women expressed annoyance, only to have someone dismiss it as "that time of the month?" This is so aggravating! While hormone imbalance isn't behind every fluctuation in our emotions, mood swings are a very real symptom.

When your progesterone dips before your period, you might feel irritable or anxious. The same goes for perimenopause and menopause when your estrogen and progesterone levels are changing. Your mood might go from happy-go-lucky to vengeful rage demon in just a few minutes! It's so frustrating! And it can take a serious toll on your relationships and quality of life.

Mood swings are one of the most common issues that I hear women blame themselves for. But how can you expect to control your emotions when your body is constantly inundated with messages (hormones are messengers, remember?) to get angry, fight, feel sad, or smile—all in a short period? That's not being fair to yourself.

Sleep

The source of sleepless nights can be tough to hone in on. A lot of issues can affect your sleep. But one thing is for sure: If you're not sleeping well, that affects your hormones. If your hormones are already out of balance, insomnia can send them into a wacky, wonky spiral.

Melatonin and cortisol can affect your sleep in big

ways. Melatonin deficiency interrupts your circadian rhythm, so your body doesn't know when it's time to sleep. Cortisol keeps your stress response activated (even if it's at a low level). You can't sleep if you're in fight-flight-or-flee mode!

Estrogen and progesterone imbalances can cause insomnia, too. A lot of pregnant women have trouble sleeping—whether because they have to get up and pee, their back hurts, their boobs are sore, their baby is kicking, or their hormones are going wild. And, of course, perimenopause and menopause are notorious for insomnia! Changing hormones can have your entire system confused about whether it feels tired. A hot flash can be so overwhelming that you wake up sweating through your sheets.

Insomnia is no joke. It affects every aspect of your life, from your moods to your concentration (we don't want you sleepy behind the wheel!), to your immune health.

Metabolism

Have you ever felt extra hungry before your period or while bleeding? That's your hormones telling you to eat! You may need more calories during certain stages of your cycle. Your body may be telling you to eat more carbs or protein (or chocolate, which could mean you need more magnesium), for example.

As you age, your hormone levels can slow down your metabolism (especially after menopause), making it tougher to lose weight. Imbalanced hormone levels can affect your insulin—and therefore, your ability to process sugar. That means your body might build up more fat (especially around your belly).

By the way, want another reason to have more orgasms? Orgasm releases the hormone oxytocin, which has a lot of wonderful, healthy, happy-making benefits—including regulating your appetite. (More on that in Chapter 6!)

SNAPSHOTS OF YOUR HORMONES THROUGH YOUR LIFE

Middle childhood and puberty

HGH keeps your body growing strong and tall at this stage of life.

Between the ages of 8 and 13, your brain triggers puberty: the pituitary gland tells your ovaries to start producing estrogen and releasing eggs. (Congratulations, girl: you've just had your first period!) Estrogen moves in and redecorates the whole place—growing your breasts, collecting a bit of fat around your hips and thighs, and giving you womanly curves. A slight rise in your androgens (including testosterone) means you grow hair under your arms and on your labia. You'll notice changes in your skin (like acne) and mood swings.

Teen years

Puberty can continue through your early teen years, though all the changes are usually in place by age 14 or 15. At that point, your menstrual cycle starts to regulate and become more predictable.

Your sex hormones are flowing at full strength now, so you'll think about sex more (sometimes a lot more!).

These hormones can also affect your mood. You might have mood swings as your hormones find their rhythm and learn to work together in harmony. Since estrogen plays a role in your serotonin levels, imbalanced estrogen levels can make teenage girls more vulnerable to mental health issues like depression and anxiety.

Your bones and muscles are building strength during your teen years, too.

Your 20s

By this time, your period should be on a predictable schedule, although it may bring some acne along with it every month—not to mention menstrual cramps that send you on a quest for the perfect painkillers.

You're fertile, and your hormones make sure your bones and muscles are strong enough to carry, nourish, and birth a baby. Your twenties are your peak fertility years. Another way your hormones support this biological drive is by making you want to get it on like crazy!

Your weight usually goes up a bit during your twenties since your metabolism and HGH are no longer working overtime to get you through childhood and puberty to the full strength of adulthood.

Your 30s

Your thirties are your strong, active mama years (even if you didn't have children and don't plan to).

You're still fertile, but your body produces fewer

hormones. Estrogen and progesterone drop around age thirty, then again in your mid-thirties. You might notice you're less interested in sex, and you might gain some weight (although it's not entirely true that your metabolism is on a steady decline after age thirty).

As your progesterone drops, your bones start to lose density faster than they can build it, and your muscles lose strength and volume more easily.

Your 40s and beyond!

Welcome to the years of The Change (*dunh-dunh-dunh*)!

Just kidding—perimenopause, menopause, and post-menopause don't have to be the horror show that society makes them out to be. Menopause isn't a hormone deficiency disease. Like puberty, the process is triggered by your brain. It's not, as most doctors believe, because your body runs out of eggs.

Perimenopause can begin as early as your thirties and as late as your mid-fifties but, for most women, it starts in their forties. It can last from 2 to 10 years. During this time, your body releases fewer eggs so you're less fertile (although some women still get pregnant in their forties). Your periods become irregular, often with long gaps between each period, and your flow may be lighter. You might start to experience hot flashes, night sweats, vaginal dryness, memory and concentration issues, and mood swings. Although, as I've mentioned, these symptoms aren't inevitable.

When you go a full year without a period, you've hit

menopause. Your baby-making days are over! You've made it through!

Most women hit this milestone around age fifty. During menopause, the symptoms of perimenopause continue. Only now, your body is producing even fewer sex hormones (estrogen and progesterone). Bones lose density with the decline in progesterone. Your sex drive might feel like a stalled car—you turn the key in the ignition and . . . nothing happens. I promise this isn't the end of your sex life! Sex after menopause can include some of the best orgasms of your life.

When your body stops making enough estrogen and progesterone, your pituitary gland tries to pick up the slack by producing more FSH (Follicle-Stimulating Hormone). A doctor can test you for FSH levels to know for sure whether you're through menopause. If you are, it's time for another congratulations! After menopause, your hormones stabilize. No more of those pesky "symptoms" that came along with menopause, like hot flashes and night sweats. You'll need to be aware of the risk of osteoporosis and cardiovascular disease, but those can be managed (I'll share how in this book). You can live the rest of your life like a goddess!

A team of geniuses on your side

Have you ever seen a sci-fi movie where a lot of smart men and women sit in a room full of computer terminals, all working together to bring a spaceship home safely? Think of those men and women as your hormones. They all have different jobs, but they all have to work together in perfect harmony to get that ship back to Earth.

Now you have a picture of how your hormones influence you throughout your life, and what happens when they're out of balance.

Next, we'll talk about one of the biggest misunderstandings in modern medicine: how estrogen affects women's health and well-being.

2

THE ESTROGEN MYTH

"Keeping your body healthy is an expression of gratitude to the whole cosmos—the trees, the clouds, everything."

— THICH NHAT HANH

P**rogestin:** Synthetic progesterone. It's meant to interact with your progesterone receptors.

In the last chapter, you learned the role that estrogen plays in your health. Think of estrogen as making you "feel like a natural woman"—with breasts, curves (thanks to fat distribution around your hips and thighs), and soft skin.

Estrogen is also involved in[4]:

- Your menstrual cycle[4]
- Supporting your uterine lining[4]
- Ovulation[4]
- Vaginal elasticity[4]
- Vaginal lubrication[4]
- Sex drive[4]
- Lactation[4]
- Cardiovascular health[4]
- Bone density[4]
- Muscle strength[4]
- Metabolism and weight[4]
- Fibroids (in the breast and uterus)[4]
- Mood[4]

In your body, estrogen and progesterone are supposed to balance one another. Estrogen alone isn't safe. Over 30 studies have shown that estrogen-only therapies increased the risk of cancer and endometrial hyperplasia (a precancerous condition where the uterine lining thickens, causing heavy and irregular bleeding, and anemia). It can also increase the risk of breast cancer, venous and pulmonary embolism, osteoporosis, and side effects like bloating, nausea, headaches, severe cramping, and irregular bleeding.[5]

ENTER PROGESTIN

When researchers and doctors saw all the risks associated with estrogen-only therapies, they remembered that estrogen occurs in the body along with progesterone. Of course! (Duh!) So they decided to add some progesterone to their hormone therapies.

The trouble is that progesterone doesn't absorb well when taken by mouth. And researchers couldn't patent progesterone, anyway. They would rather work with a synthetic version they could make a lot of money with. So they created progestin—synthetic progesterone.

Hallelujah! This was surely the answer they'd been looking for!

When the pill was developed in the 1950s, it included a combination of synthetic estrogens and synthetic progestin. Initial trials were flawed, to say the least—trials were done in secret on populations of poor women in Puerto Rico, who weren't informed about the risks of the drug they were taking. The pills included ridiculously high levels of hormones which caused serious side effects, including blood clots, depression, and nausea . . . but the women who came forward to report these side effects were ignored. Even the three women who died during the trial were ignored.

The pill was eventually sold to the public as a way to prevent pregnancy and regulate menstruation.[6]

These days, the pill is available in lower doses of hormones—but even the lowest doses aren't safe for all women. The combined pill (containing both estrogen and progestin) doesn't regulate menstruation. It completely *stops menstruation*. You only bleed each month because you stop taking the hormones for a week.[7]

Hear me, ladies: *This is not a period!* It's withdrawal bleeding!

Plus, the pill is associated with risks of coronary artery disease, breast cancer, high blood pressure, and more.[7]

If you've ever been on the pill (or any hormonal birth control), you might be familiar with the side effects. They can include nausea, vomiting, headaches, breast tenderness, weight gain, mood swings, changes in sex drive, blood clots, and vaginitis. If you've ever had asthma, migraines, epilepsy, or heart disease, the pill can make your symptoms worse.[7]

There are also implications for mental health. Many women aren't aware that the pill causes structural changes in their brains. It can shrink your hypothalamus by as much as 6%,[8] raise your cortisol, and lower your testosterone. (Higher stress and a lower sex drive? That's the opposite of what women want!) The pill reduces your serotonin and alters your neurotransmitters in a way that makes you more likely to develop depression or anxiety.[9,10]

Hormonal birth control and all its side effects still aren't fully understood.

But that hasn't stopped science from marching blindly forward.

INTRODUCING HRT

As they saw it, researchers had solved women's desire for birth control. Now they turned their attention to a whole new group of women complaining about hormone issues:

menopausal women! Enter the development of HRT (Hormone Replacement Therapy).

Seeing as estrogen declines during menopause, it makes sense that doctors believe supplementing estrogen must be the key to helping women. But that's wrong. Here's a quote from Leslie Kenton, author of *Passage to Power: Natural Menopause Revolution:*

> "Everybody who is anybody will tell you that menopause is an estrogen-deficiency disease and that you will need to take more estrogen as you approach mid-life. What may surprise you is this: not only is most of such commonly given advice on menopause wrong, a great deal of it can be positively dangerous.[11]

In 2022, Dr. Bruce Dorr also wrote about the misunderstandings surrounding menopause. He pointed out that over 30 symptoms can pop up due to hormonal imbalances during this time in a woman's life, but most doctors don't connect them with menopause. Dr. Dorr wrote:

> "Over the years, I have treated female patients referred to cardiologists for irregular heartbeats, endocrinologists for weight gain, and marriage counselors for vaginal dryness and loss of libido. None of these specialists had prescribed effective treatments, because changes in

hormone levels were not identified as the root cause...

"... Consider also that in the United States, 80% of medical residents reported feeling 'barely comfortable' discussing or treating menopause, and only 20% of OB/GYN residency programs provide menopause training, mostly through elective courses . . . There has always been a lack of research into women's health, and we are just now starting to realize how much we don't know."[12]

Even today, doctors just don't "get" menopause! Most of them are barely comfortable discussing it. I would think their common sense would tell them that when a woman over 40 has a symptom, it might have something to do with her baseline hormone levels fluctuating like crazy. But nope! Most doctors' minds don't even go there.

The situation was even worse in the 1950s and '60s. But they wanted to help their patients, and pharmaceutical companies swore the answer was HRT. So, with limited understanding, doctors started prescribing HRT for menopausal women left and right.

One of the most popular forms of synthetic estrogen in HRT is called "Premarin." Take a look at the word and see if you can guess what it's made from: Pre-mar-in.

If you jokingly guessed "pregnant mare urine . . ." you're

right! (Oh, how I wish you were wrong!) That's truly what Premarin is made from: the urine of pregnant mares.[13] Just what a woman's body needs! Pregnant mares produce 10 different types of estrogen. But a woman's body naturally produces only three types. It's no wonder our bodies have trouble making sense of all these unfamiliar, unnatural forms of estrogen!

HRT has all the same risks as the pill. But it's given at lower doses than the pill, so the side effects are often more subtle and slower to show up.

Are you starting to catch on to the fact that medical science's "solutions" to women's health are actually creating more problems?

Synthetic hormones wreak havoc!

I'm not being dramatic with that headline! Synthetic estrogen and progestin are flat-out not good for your body. Some of the most serious complications include cardiovascular disease and breast cancer.

Let's look at some research studies.

Cardiovascular disease

Some sources (including doctors and pharmaceutical companies) might tell you that using estrogen—either alone or in combination with synthetic progestins—can decrease the risk of cardiovascular diseases.

Don't you believe it!

In one study published by the University of California at San Diego,[14] researchers worked with 16,608 women between the ages of 50 and 79. They all had an intact uterus.

One group was given a placebo, and the other was given HRT that contained synthetic estrogen and progestin. Researchers wanted to be sure these pills were safe and effective. But after 5.2 years, they had to call off the trial. Compared to the placebo group, women in the trial group had:

- 29% more CHD events. (Coronary heart disease, the #1 cause of death in the United States, occurs when the arteries can't deliver enough oxygen-rich blood to the heart.)
- 41% more strokes. (A stroke occurs when the blood supply to the brain gets restricted. When your brain can't get enough oxygen and nutrients, its cells begin dying within minutes.)
- 22% higher rates of cardiovascular disease.
- 26% more invasive breast cancer.
- 2-fold higher rates of VTE. (Venous thromboembolism, which means blood clots form in your veins. Two common types of VTE are deep vein thrombosis and pulmonary embolism.)

Yikes! The study determined: *"Overall health risks exceeded benefits* from use of combined estrogen plus progestin for an average 5.2-year follow-up among healthy postmenopausal US women."

Another study, also published by UC San Diego,[15] came to similar alarming conclusions. This was another randomized, double-blind placebo trial that included 10,739 women. One group was given a placebo, and the other was given a synthetic "conjugated equine estrogen . . ." which means hormones made from pregnant mare pee (like Premarin). Once again, they were forced to end the trial early.

Compared to the placebo group, the women in the trial experienced:

- 39% more strokes.
- 33% more VTE.
- 12% higher total cardiovascular disease events (including stroke).

Both studies concluded that the risks outweigh the benefits of these "treatments." I couldn't agree more!

These studies only involved postmenopausal women. But the risks are high for younger women on hormonal therapies, too. Women taking the combined pill have:

- 4-fold higher risk of VTE (VTE risk is even higher for pregnant women, even if they're not on the pill).
- 20–30% higher risk of breast cancer.
- Higher blood pressure (leading to an increased risk of stroke and heart disease).

Breast cancer
In the United States, 1 in 8 women will develop breast

cancer in their lives.[16] Researchers are studying it like crazy, trying to understand what's going on, how to prevent it, and how to cure it. But studies about hormones and breast cancer keep coming up with mixed results. This has scientists confused.

I don't feel confused about it. My common sense tells me that synthetic hormones are associated with hormone-related cancers.

One thing researchers are sure of is that the combined pill, which blends estrogens and synthetic progestin, does raise your breast cancer risk. The longer you're on the pill, the more your risk creeps up . . . and up . . . and up.

A 2004 French study compared 98,997 women born between 1925 and 1950.[17] Some of the women were on different forms of HRT, and others were not. Researchers followed their health journeys for nearly six years. They found that in all forms of HRT where estrogens were combined with synthetic progestins, breast cancer risk went up:

> *"Even short durations of exposure were associated with significantly increased risks when estrogens were combined with synthetic progestins."[17]*

These findings show up again and again in similar studies.

The most impressive one may just be the "Million Women Study." It involved 1,084,110 UK women aged 50 to

64 years. They shared information about their health histories and HRT use. Researchers kept up with them for about five years (between 1996 and 2001), taking note of cancer and death rates.[18] Here are some of their findings:

- Current users of HRT were more likely to develop breast cancer than women who had never used it, or women who stopped using it.[18]
- The longer a woman used HRT, the higher her risk.[18]
- The risk was high for women on estrogen-only products, women on tibolone (a synthetic form of progesterone), and women on combined estrogen-progestin. No form of HRT was risk-free. But the "risk was substantially greater for estrogen-progestogen than for other types of HRT."[18]
- There are different types of synthetic estrogens and progestins. The risk of cancer is high for all types.[18]
- Oral, transdermal, and implant methods of estrogen-only products were all high risk.[18]
- Over 10 years of estrogen-only HRT use, about 5 additional cases of breast cancer for every 1,000 women were reported.[18]
- Over 10 years of estrogen-progestogen HRT use, about 19 additional cases of breast cancer for every 1,000 women were reported.[18]

- "Use of HRT by women aged 50 to 64 years in the UK over the past decade has resulted in an estimated 20,000 extra breast cancers, 15,000 associated with estrogen-progestogen; the extra deaths cannot yet be reliably estimated."[18]

How can doctors still recommend this treatment for women in good conscience?

In the studies I mentioned, estrogen-only therapies came out looking a little better than combined estrogen-progestin versions. But that doesn't mean estrogen gets off scot-free. Estrogen-only therapies were still associated with risk.

Your risks go up if you're overweight. That's because estrogen is stored in the fatty tissue of your body (called adipose tissue), including your breasts.[19] This tissue both stores and produces estrogen. That means the more fat you have, the more estrogen you have. Did you know that a fat postmenopausal woman produces more estrogen than a thin, younger woman? And remember that as you age, your metabolism slows down (thanks a lot, HGH!), meaning your body holds on to that estrogen-rich fat longer.

While premenopausal fat women have lower rates of breast cancer than thinner women, this completely flip-flops once you hit menopause—which is when most cases of breast cancer occur. Postmenopausal women who are overweight have a 20–60% higher risk than thin women of developing breast cancers.[20]

I'll also mention xenoestrogens here since your body

treats those as estrogen (it doesn't know what else to do with these confusing lab-made chemicals). That skyrockets the amount of estrogen accumulating in your body! These xenoestrogens are even leading to higher rates of breast cancer among men, as they grow men's breast tissue (a condition called gynecomastia). Men also have to deal with a higher prostate cancer risk.

Like with the studies on cardiovascular disease, the breast cancer research I mentioned focused on menopausal women. But the risk is still present for women in their childbearing years. If you're taking the pill, your risk goes up by 20–30%.[21,22]

Even more havoc!

Cardiovascular disease and breast cancer are two of the biggest complications of using HRT or the pill. But they're far from the only issues![23,24]

Your risk goes up for:

- Blood clots.
- Heart attacks.
- Liver tumors.
- Gallstones.
- Ectopic pregnancy.
- Osteoporosis.
- Thyroid disorders. (The rate of thyroid prescriptions for women over 40 is now surpassing heart medications.)

- Anxiety and depression. (So much for hoping synthetic hormones can help balance your moods!)

Your body's endocrine system orchestrates a complex, holistic process, and your hormones all work together to maintain balance.

Synthetic hormones are endocrine disruptors (there, I said it!). Introducing a foreign hormone into your delicate biological system disrupts the work of all of the others. Hundreds of physiological processes are thrown out of whack.

Here's an example of how: Your body has specific receptors for your natural hormones. Estrogen binds with your estrogen receptors, progesterone binds with your progesterone receptors, etc. You would think that synthetic progestin should be designed to bind with the same receptors as your natural hormone . . . but you'd be wrong! It actually binds with a whole host of receptors throughout your body, sending confusing signals through your system.[25]

Synthetic hormones stop your body from producing its natural hormones, which can confuse your body into thinking it's going through menopause. Plus, as your body works overtime to metabolize the high doses of hormones flooding your system, your essential nutrients get depleted—nutrients like magnesium, essential fatty acids, vitamins C and E, and various B vitamins. Your body needs these exact nutrients to keep your hormones balanced! The harder your system works, the more overwhelmed it gets, and the less capable it is of doing its job.

Synthetic hormones disrupt your body

They quite literally change your body. But their effects can be so slow-moving and subtle, that it's not always clear they're working. That means you can be on them for a long time, and you won't realize the damage they've done until it's too late. All the while, they've been quietly transforming your body in ways you didn't sign up for and don't want.

I want you to understand that you don't have to take these risks with your health. You don't have to rely on the pill during your childbearing years, and you can age gracefully without turning to HRT. (Your menopause is not a deficiency disease that desperately has to be treated so your body won't weaken, shrivel up, and fall apart!)

In the next chapter, you'll learn about the role that your natural progesterone plays in your health—and the one product I recommend to virtually every person who comes to me with a hormone imbalance.

SARA'S STORY

One day, I noticed a woman checking out natural products for babies in my vitamin store. She was frowning a little, as people sometimes do when trying to decide between a few products. But I was helping another customer and she left without buying anything. Oh well! Maybe she would come back.

She was back a few days later, this time lingering in the aisle for pregnancy and motherhood. She had a little baby, maybe a month old, swaddled up in a fancy stroller with all the bells and whistles (a cup holder, pockets for her purse and phone—this thing had it all!), and she rolled the stroller gently back and forth while she read the labels on several products. One of my coworkers offered her help, but she said, "I'm good, thanks." Again, she left without buying anything.

The third time I saw her come in was the next week, and she'd brought her little one again. I was determined to talk to her this time. She clearly needed something, but maybe she wasn't sure what. For whatever reason, she was reluctant to ask for help with it. The aura of loneliness that seemed to hang around her like a heavy cloak broke my heart a little.

I approached and said, "Can I help you find anything?"

As I expected, she politely declined. But I wouldn't be put off so easily. Babies are always a great conversation starter. "Aww, look at this little guy! He's adorable! What's his name?"

"Cameron." She smiled, but there was a distant quality to it. Talking about her baby hadn't lit her up at all. I began to suspect I might know her problem.

"I've seen you in here a few times, little Cameron," I said to her baby, who was fast asleep. "I've helped a lot of new moms like yours. Some of them need help with breastfeeding, some can't sleep, and some are just struggling to adjust to being a mom."

Now I had Mama's attention. She smiled politely, engaging more with me. "Actually . . . maybe you can help me?"

"Let's find out," I said. "What's going on?"

"Well . . . I'm not exactly sure. I had him over a month ago. The pregnancy was healthy, the birth was difficult but ultimately fine. But now . . . I don't know. Something is off."

"Can you describe what's off?"

She sighed. "Everything. I'm not sleeping, even though I'm tired all the time—and I don't think it's all his fault." She looked at Cameron, who didn't seem to have trouble in the sleep department. "I can't concentrate. The other day I forgot to turn off the water after washing my hands. What the hell, right? I keep telling my husband it's a good thing I'm on maternity leave because I wouldn't get any work done. And my emotions are just all over the place. I feel disconnected for hours, and then all of a sudden I'm crying about nothing."

I nodded. "That's got to be confusing and frustrating. Can I ask you a question?"

"Go ahead."

"How do you feel about being a mom?"

She took a deep breath, and her eyes filled with helplessness. "I haven't even told my husband this." She began to open up. She told me her name was Sara and, over the course of our chat, she admitted, "I wanted Cameron so much. I was so thrilled to be pregnant with him, but now . . . I don't feel like his mother. Sometimes it feels like I'm caring for another woman's child. Is there something wrong with me?

Am I a bad mom?" Her eyes welled with tears, but she willed them away. I could tell she spent a lot of energy trying to be strong.

"Not at all!" I reassured her. "Your experience is actually pretty common. I think you're experiencing postpartum depression."

"Baby Blues?" she said, a little skeptical. "My doctor told me not to worry about that. He said my hormones would just stabilize naturally."

I kind of wanted to wring her doctor's neck. Politely, of course. "It's a little more than 'Baby Blues.'"

I explained how a woman's hormones, especially her progesterone, run high throughout her pregnancy. But after the birth, those hormone levels drop—fast and low. The hormone fluctuations in a woman's body can affect her thyroid function, HPA axis (the relationship between the hypothalamus, pituitary, and amygdala, where these glands communicate with each other to produce healthy hormone levels), and even her genetic expression in certain cases.

Some women's hormones do stabilize naturally. For other women, the sudden hormone drop is like falling off a cliff. It's especially prevalent in women who struggled with depression or anxiety before pregnancy.

"This isn't the kind of thing you can wish away with positive affirmations," I said. "It's a real form of depression. And that's not always easy to treat naturally."

I gave her a topical progesterone cream to help her hormone levels return to normal. She didn't want to take pharmaceuticals (though she didn't feel like a mom, she was still trying to make the best decisions for her baby). So I talked about a few natural ways to get through depression, like using St. John's wort, getting her oxytocin up with sex and masturbation, making sure to eat well, and getting a little gentle exercise in her routine.

"Let's start with those changes and the progesterone cream," I said. "Come see me again in a month, and we'll go from there."

Over the next six months, Sara and I got to know each other. We worked together to get her hormones back to healthy levels, and she eventually fell in love with little Cameron. I saw her smile more often, and she began to get more (and better) rest. Sara began to truly enjoy being a mother ... and even talking about her next baby.

3

THE ANSWER: NATURAL PROGESTERONE

"He who has health has hope; and he who has hope has everything."

— ARABIAN PROVERB

So far, I've talked about estrogen and how doctors don't really understand it. You've also learned that estrogen occurs naturally alongside progesterone and that synthetic progestins fall seriously short of replacing your natural hormone. (That's putting it politely!)

Now it's time to talk about progesterone itself: what it is, how it affects your cycles and your system, and what happens when your progesterone is too low.

And yes—you'll learn about a bunch of supplements, herbs, and products that make synthetic hormones totally unnecessary . . . including the one product I recommend for everybody who comes to me for advice (I'm talking younger women, older women, men, and even children!).

PROGESTERONE'S ROLE IN YOUR BODY

Your body produces three types of estrogen. That makes estrogen more like a "class" of hormones.

Your body only produces one type of progesterone. It's called . . . (*drumroll!*) . . . progesterone. Think of progesterone as a "class" of hormones, with just a single member in the class. It's the one, the only.

But progesterone is also the precursor of a whole host of other hormones. It's involved in creating testosterone and corticosteroids, which are critical for things like your sex drive, blood sugar and electrolyte balance, blood pressure, stress response, and survival in the face of imminent danger (you can't run from a lion if your hormones don't activate your stress response).[26]

After your body ovulates, a temporary endocrine gland is formed. It's called the corpus luteum. Your corpus luteum creates progesterone, which has the big job of making sure your uterine lining is thick and nutrient-rich enough to support a fertilized egg. It also prevents muscle contractions in the uterus.

If you don't get pregnant, your corpus luteum says, "I

guess I'm not needed this time. See you next month!" And it breaks down and dissolves.

If you do get pregnant, your body invites progesterone to take over the entire place. It brings in all of its luggage and moves into the master bedroom. It stocks your kitchen with its favorite foods and cooks big, elaborate meals. It redecorates and makes itself at home. How? Your corpus luteum sticks around, making more of the hormone to keep your body in peak pregnancy condition. Your placenta forms around week 12, and it starts producing progesterone too. It produces so much that your corpus luteum is finally allowed to dissolve.

High levels of progesterone prevent ovulation, so you don't get pregnant while you're already pregnant. Progesterone also grows your breasts, getting them ready for lactation. When you're pregnant, your body produces the hormone HCG (Human Chorionic Gonadotropin), which signals your ovaries to keep producing progesterone. It also nurtures the fetus.

Basically, your body pulls out all the stops to keep your progesterone levels nice and high—up to 10 times higher than when you're not pregnant. Your progesterone should stay high right up through to when you give birth.[27]

After menopause, your progesterone levels drop . . . sometimes as much as 99%. Even if your estrogen levels also drop, they won't drop as low as your progesterone. That means you're now estrogen dominant.

But wait, there's more!

Most doctors won't tell you much more about progesterone than that. They think of progesterone as an ovulation and pregnancy hormone. They're not educated on the role it plays throughout your life—through menopause and beyond.

They won't mention that progesterone is also important for your sex drive, menstrual regulation, thyroid, brain, nerve cells, energy levels, corticosteroid production, your ability to manage stress (like surgery, trauma, or personal loss), blood pressure, stabilizing your glucose levels, preventing arthritis and chronic pain, fluid retention and weight gain, and anti-aging (since it's important for collagen production). It's even a must-have for building strong bones.

PROGESTERONE AND YOUR BONES

Dr. John Lee, author of *Hormone Balance Made Simple*, has done a lot of research on progesterone and bone density. He was even able to identify progesterone receptors on osteoblast cells (these are your bone-building cells). Contrary to popular belief, estrogen isn't the bone-building hormone. *Progesterone is.*[27,28]

I first learned this truth years ago. At one of my vitamin stores, so many women came in with osteoporosis that I decided to make a big investment: a bone density testing machine. It was called the "Heel Ultrasound," and at the time, it was considered pretty accurate. (It's not considered accurate anymore.) Every time I tested my bones with this machine, it said that I had osteopenia. Well, I didn't want brittle bones! I was too young to start cracking and breaking!

My customers told me about this new wonder drug called Fosamax. It was supposed to be the best stuff to prevent bone loss that science could cook up in a lab.

Hmm . . . a pharmaceutical, huh? Would it be right for me? I dove into my research.

What I found made it all too clear: *no*. This was not right for me. It wasn't right for *anyone*! Fosamax had too many nasty potential side effects . . . including burning your esophagus! Patients had to stand up while taking the drug and couldn't lie down for at least half an hour, so it wouldn't reflux and burn their esophagus! Sounds like a miracle cure to me (*not*)! Sure, it helped create new bone, but the new bone was porous and brittle. So brittle that another side effect was . . . (*wait for it*) . . . femur fractures! That's right—the bone density drug could cause the strongest, largest bone in your body to fracture.

Sometimes the audacity of drug companies still amazes me.

Needless to say, I skipped the Fosamax. My research led me to Dr. Lee's work on progesterone and bone density, as well as other studies that corroborated his findings.

Common knowledge says that postmenopausal women naturally lose bone density—at a "Whoa, Nelly!" rate of 1.5% per year. And that this bone loss is due to decreasing estrogen levels. But in a three-year study of 63 postmenopausal women with osteoporosis, women using progesterone cream saw significant bone mass density increases. On average, they saw 7–8% more density in the first year. In the second year, the increases were 4–5%. In the third year, the increases were 3–4%. (So the biggest gains were during the first year, with decreasing benefits each consecutive year.)[28]

Dr. Lee believes that using natural progesterone cream (along with a healthy diet and lifestyle) can not only stop osteoporosis but can actually reverse it—even in women over 70!

As for me, I used progesterone cream and had my bones tested by a more reliable method years later. They were nice and strong.[28]

WHAT CAUSES UNBALANCED PROGESTERONE?

If your progesterone is too high . . . don't worry about it! There are no known negative consequences for having high progesterone.

If your progesterone is low, it's a different story. In that case, an avalanche of problems can overwhelm your physical and emotional health.

Low progesterone can happen if you don't ovulate regularly because your corpus luteum doesn't form. Thyroid problems (which have become rampant in Western societies) are also big culprits. If you have hypothyroidism, your thyroid isn't producing enough hormones to properly regulate your endocrine system.[26]

If you struggle with anxiety or depression, your body may be chronically flooded with stress hormones. Cortisol steals the natural substances that your body uses to make progesterone. Hey, if you're fighting for your life (or if your anxiety *thinks you are*), you don't have the bandwidth to worry about reproduction or maintaining your body's delicate hormone balance. You've got to survive! That's just fine if you're running from a bear or jumping out of the path of a crazy driver . . . but it's a big problem if all your body's resources are chronically funneled to survival.

If your cholesterol is too low, or if your pituitary gland makes too much prolactin, your body may also interrupt your progesterone production.[26]

And, of course, if you're estrogen dominant, that means your progesterone levels just can't keep up with your outrageous, sky-high estrogen levels.

I'm going to make a big, bold statement here, and say that most people in Western societies (women for sure, but also men and children) have too much estrogen in their systems. Our lives revolve around endocrine-disrupting, xenoestrogen-laden products. You can try to live a natural, "crunchy," and toxin-free lifestyle . . . but it's impossible to get away from xenoestrogens. You'll learn more about them in Chapter 4.

SIGNS YOU MAY HAVE LOW PROGESTERONE

If you ask your doctor to test your estrogen and progesterone levels, she'll probably do a blood test. The results might come back showing that you're completely normal and have nothing to worry about (even if you *know* something is wrong).

That's because a blood test isn't the best way to identify low progesterone.

A blood test is a snapshot of your blood hormone levels at one specific time of day. It tells you nothing about the history of your hormones. What were they doing yesterday or last month?

To identify low progesterone (or high estrogen), you'll want to have your saliva and urine tested. This is something I often do for my clients, especially with hair. I take several samples of their hair (from as close to the root as possible) and send them off to a lab for analysis. This paints a picture of their hormone fluctuations over a longer period of time instead of just a few hours one morning.

Just as a reminder, I'm not a doctor. I'm a woman trained in functional nutrition who has worked in the natural health industry for over 20 years. But my experience working with hundreds of women has shown me that low progesterone has a long laundry list of symptoms.

So if this list looks crazy long, that's because it is! I would never pad the list with extra symptoms. (In fact, I might be leaving some things out!) I just want to impress upon you the multifaceted role that progesterone plays in your body. If it's out of balance, that's going to have a cascade of negative effects on your health. It can manifest itself in so many ways.

You probably won't have all of these symptoms. You might currently have just one or two. But please understand that if you do have a few, your risk goes up for the others. For example, if your periods are irregular and very low flow, you're at risk for infertility, uterine fibroids, low libido, and more. If you're having hot flashes, you're at risk for osteoporosis, thyroid issues, and more. Your symptoms might seem unrelated, like irregular periods and insomnia. Everything on this list is interconnected because your body is a holistic, unified being. What affects one part of you, affects the whole of you.

Some of these symptoms are more directly related to estrogen dominance, rather than low progesterone. If your progesterone is low, then estrogen naturally becomes your dominant hormone. This comes with its own host of problems (PCOS, tender breasts, PMS, weight gain, etc.), which we'll talk about in more depth in Chapter 4. That said, it's not usually relevant to isolate whether you're dealing with low progesterone or dominant estrogen, because the two conditions go hand in hand.

Okay, I've gotten the relevant disclaimers out of the way! Here's a list of symptoms indicating that you may have low progesterone:

- **Anovulation** – If you're not ovulating or having a period, your progesterone is low.[26,27]
- **Infertility** – Fertility and pregnancy depend on healthy progesterone.[26,27]
- **Irregular periods** – A hallmark sign![26,27]
- **Heavy periods (aka "flooding")** – Your uterine lining will thicken, and thicken, and thicken until it feels like you're bleeding constantly and dropping clots of blood.[26,27]
- **Osteoporosis** – If progesterone isn't around to build your bones, they'll grow brittle and weak.[26,27]
- **Nerve issues & brain fog** – Progesterone helps create the myelin sheath, which forms around your nerves (including nerves in your brain and spinal cord).[26,27]
- **Arthritis & chronic pain** – Because progesterone is involved in collagen, bone building, and nerve health, its absence can lead to joint issues and chronic pain.[26,27]
- **Facial hair growth & thinning hair** – Your androgens (male hormones like testosterone) can get out of balance without progesterone. That means you'll get male symptoms of facial hair growth and thinning hair.[26,27]
- **Sagging, loose skin** – Progesterone supports collagen production. Without that, your skin loses elasticity and can't repair itself as fast.[26,27]

- **Low libido** – Progesterone helps you get horny! Without it, you won't want to get it on.[26,27]
- **Depression & anxiety** – Progesterone keeps your GABA receptors and serotonin healthy. These are neurotransmitters involved in calming your stress response.[26,27]
- **Insomnia** – If progesterone isn't around to activate those relaxing neurotransmitters, sleep can be hard to come by.[26,27]
- **Fibrocystic breasts** – Estrogen dominance can cause lumpy, tender breasts. These lumps are typically benign but can cause a lot of discomfort and stress.[26,27]
- **Uterine fibroids** – Just like breast fibroids, too much estrogen can lead to uterine fibroids. Again, these are typically non-cancerous.[26,27]
- **Fluid retention and weight gain** – If you ever feel bloated before your period, that's because your estrogen levels are higher. If your estrogen is dominant all the time, you'll retain more water. When it comes to fat itself (adipose tissue), a little is okay. But too much estrogen can lead to more fat, which then creates more estrogen, which then creates more fat . . . you get the idea. You need some progesterone to balance that out.[26,27]
- **Hot flashes & night sweats** – Doctors have no idea what causes hot flashes. You go to them with a very clear symptom, and all they can do is shrug

and say "That just happens sometimes when you get older. It's inevitable." But no. It's not. You just need to balance your estrogen with more progesterone.[26,27]
- **Headaches & migraines** – Any hormone fluctuation can lead to a headache, but if you're dealing with headaches along with other issues on this list, low progesterone could be to blame.[26,27]
- **PMS** – Even supposedly "standard" PMS symptoms, like cramps and mood swings, are often caused by low progesterone.[26,27]
- **Thyroid issues** – Your thyroid is directly related to your overall hormone health. Thyroid issues can affect your progesterone, and vice versa.[26,27]

If you think you have a few of these symptoms but you're not sure, I urge you to err on the side of caution—especially if you're currently on the pill or HRT. As I've mentioned, sometimes the effects of hormone treatments can take a while to show up. During the months that you're wondering whether your pharmaceuticals are working, they're quietly changing your body. That means a small symptom can quickly escalate into a big problem . . . or a handful of big problems.

Low progesterone can wreak havoc at any stage of your life. But during pregnancy, it's a serious danger. Complications can include spotting and even miscarriage. And even if you're not pregnant, serious risks include uterine or breast cancer.

CAN YOU REPLACE PROGESTERONE WITH SYNTHETIC PROGESTIN?

Nope. There's no competition between the two. One is progesterone, while the other is "franken-gesterone."

One is naturally produced by your body. Women and men both produce it, though men require less than women. (Men need a little progesterone for healthy sperm development and testosterone levels.) Progesterone locks into specific receptors throughout your body. They're called progesterone receptors (imagine that!).

Synthetic progestin, on the other hand, is made by mad scientists in labs from the urine of pregnant mares. Contrary to what many women have been told by their doctors (who should know better), it's *not identical to your natural hormone.* So it's no surprise that your system doesn't quite know how to make sense of it. Your body sees this strange, foreign substance and says to itself, "Well, it's a hormone . . . and it looks a little like progesterone, I guess?"

You might think the synthetic hormone interacts with your progesterone receptors, right? That's what it's meant to do. Well, you'd be right and wrong! Because this trickster interacts with *a lot of different hormone receptors* all throughout your body.[25] That's why it sends your entire system haywire!

JOSIE'S STORY

Zarina and I had been friends for 20 years. She knew about my work at the vitamin store and sometimes asked me about natural health and supplements. I was always happy to help! Her family sometimes felt like my own.

One day, Zarina brought her beautiful, accomplished, 19-year-old daughter Josie into my store. Josie had sun-kissed skin and brown hair streaked with natural highlights. She was incredibly fit and had been a high school athlete. Her shoulders were squared, and her chin lifted with confidence.

After we finished hugging hello, Zarina said, "Liz, we actually came to see you for some advice."

"Of course! You know I love helping you!"

"Well, this question isn't actually for me. It's for Josie. She has some questions about fertility."

"Sure! What's up, kiddo?"

With her characteristic sunny smile, Josie said, "You know my boyfriend and I have been dating for a long time, right? Well, we want to get married next year."

"Wow, congratulations!" I said. "He's a wonderful guy!"

"Thank you!" she beamed. "And we want to have a big family. Lots of kids!"

"Excellent! You're going to make a great mom!" She would, too! She was incredibly loving and fun, and she also knew how to set boundaries.

But Josie's smile dimmed a bit. She looked concerned. "The thing is, I'm not sure I'm fertile."

"Why is that?"

"Because I don't have periods. Or when I do, they're really few and far between, and the flow is super light. Is there anything I can do to boost my fertility?"

I said, "Well, let's back up. Your fertility might not even be the issue. I think it might be your period."

"But if I'm not bleeding, doesn't that mean I'm not ovulating?"

"Not necessarily," I explained. "It's true that ovulation and periods do go hand in hand for women with healthy hormones. But if your hormones are off, the whole thing can go topsy-turvy! For example, some women don't ovulate, yet they still bleed. (That's obviously not a healthy period, it's called 'abnormal uterine bleeding.') And other women *do* ovulate but then *don't* have a period. I have a hunch that you might be one of them."

"So if I'm ovulating, but not bleeding, does that mean I can get pregnant?"

"No, you'd still want a healthy period for pregnancy to occur."

The poor girl looked so confused.

"There's still hope!" I said. "Let me ask you this: how often do you exercise, and what do you usually eat?"

I thought I knew the answers to this but wanted to confirm it with her. She explained that she exercised every day for a few hours, and yes, she ate tons of veggies. She loved lean proteins, low to no carbs, low to no cholesterol, and no sugar. At first glance, this sounds like a prescription-perfect diet for a lot of people. It's so healthy! But a lifestyle this extreme isn't healthy for most women—especially women who exercise as much as Josie did.

"Okay, I think I know what the problem is," I said. "You don't have enough body fat and cholesterol."

"Body fat and cholesterol?" Josie frowned. "But I thought I didn't want those things?"

"You don't want too much of them, that's true. But too little means your body can't produce the hormones required to ovulate. That's called anovulation: when you're not ovulating. And your body also can't form a healthy uterine lining for your fertilized egg to latch onto."

"But I'm not underweight," she said.

"That's because muscles are heavier than fat. So it's possible for the scale to say you're at the right weight when really you still don't have enough fat."

Understanding dawned in her eyes. "I've never thought about it like that."

Josie wasn't alone. Many female athletes fall into this situation. Athletic coaches who train young women should treat a girl's period as a marker for her health. If she's not bleeding, then she's training too hard and eating too lightly. It's a form of malnutrition. Coaches have to find a balance between training hard and ensuring their girls are healthy. Anovulation also happens to women with anorexia.

As one study put it:

> *"A high proportion of well-trained dancers and*

> *athletes have amenorrhea ["amenorrhea" means you're not having periods], though weight may be in the normal range, since muscles are heavy (80% water, compared to 5–10% water in adipose tissue). The amenorrhea is usually reversible with weight gain, decreased exercise or both. The amenorrhea is due to hypothalamic dysfunction; the pituitary-ovary axis is intact, suggesting that this type of amenorrhea is adaptive, preventing an unsuccessful pregnancy outcome. Evidence is presented that the high percentage of body fat (26–28%) in mature women is necessary for regular ovulatory cycles."[29]*

That study showed that for many women who don't have periods, the hypothalamus isn't able to do its job. The body understands that it's not in a good position to carry a healthy baby to term (not without seriously endangering the mother), so the body responds by shutting down ovulation altogether. It's the body trying to conserve its resources.

I further explained to Josie that progesterone and estrogen are produced from cholesterol. "So while you don't want your cholesterol getting too high, you definitely don't want it too low, either." After talking more, I helped her see that she could include healthy, fat-rich foods (like salmon, nuts, and avocados) in her diet without actually getting fat. "I'm confident we can get your periods going again if you change your diet, add some nutrients and herbs, and just exercise a little less."

Josie was all smiles again. "I can definitely do that! How long will it take?"

"If you stick with the program, you should start seeing changes in three months. But don't try getting pregnant just yet. Let's make sure your periods are regular and healthy first."

"Okay," she said. "I don't need to get pregnant this year. I'm definitely thinking long term. We want a big family."

"Wonderful!" I said. "I'd be honored to help you get there!"

And get there she did. One year later, Josie's wonderful boyfriend became her wonderful husband. A short time after that, she had her first child. Today, Josie is a happily married woman with five beautiful children.

BOOST YOUR NATURAL PROGESTERONE

You have a lot of options that don't involve dosing yourself up on synthetic hormones.

Some foods, herbs, and supplements can boost your body's natural progesterone. So why aren't they prescribed by your doctor? Simple: they can't be patented, so pharmaceutical companies can't make money off of them. That's why your doctor won't know much (if anything) about them. If you ask her, she'll most likely say she doesn't know much, or that natural methods haven't been proven to work.

She may have looked at a few studies or read some literature from pharmaceutical companies, but she hasn't seen progesterone-boosting methods in action.

In some regions, such as Japan and South American countries, hot flashes are so uncommon that *there isn't even a word for them!* Women in these countries tend to have diets that are rich in natural sources of hormones, including progesterone and phytoestrogens—Mexican wild yams and soybeans are some of the best examples. (But don't run to the grocery store and fill your fridge with yummy soybeans. Soy sold in the United States is a different type which will increase your estrogen. That's the opposite of what you want!)

In regions like this, menopause isn't seen as a time when women lose their energy and health along with their fertility. It's not a medical condition that needs treatment. Instead, it's a natural phase of a woman's life when she comes into a higher level of her own power. All the energy that was used for childbearing can now go to other things.

You'll find specific suggestions for what foods to eat and what to avoid in Chapter 6, along with supplements and herbs that can seriously transform your health. But one product is so powerful, I want to introduce you to it right away.

The #1 product to start using today!

I won't bury the lede: it's natural progesterone cream or wild yam cream!

I recommend this miracle supplement to just about

everyone who comes my way. Wild yams contain a steroid hormone that's similar to your progesterone. You can get a cream made from wild yams, or just use progesterone cream.

The estrogen-dominant body soaks this goodness up like water in a desert! It supports your body to metabolize and flush out excess estrogen. This includes all those xenoestrogens that you've absorbed from using harsh cleaning products, drinking out of plastic bottles, eating out of plastic leftover containers, and sleeping on sheets laundered with chemical detergents.

I suggest everyone be on this stuff! Menopausal women, fertile women, women who aren't bleeding, women who have gut issues, women who have osteoporosis, and more. I even suggest it for some men and children.

Clearing up the mystery

I hope I've cleared up some of the mysteries surrounding progesterone. I understand how frustrating it can be when you're dealing with symptoms (some of which might not seem directly related to your hormones at all). Your doctor may say that nothing can be done, or that she isn't sure what's going on . . . or that synthetic hormones are the answer to your prayers.

But you have natural options.

In the next chapter, we'll talk more about the "sister condition" that always appears with low progesterone: estrogen dominance.

Now go get some progesterone cream from your local health food store!

4

ESTROGEN DOMINANCE

"To keep the body in good health is a duty ... otherwise we shall not be able to keep the mind strong and clear."

— BUDDHA

We haven't met, but I'm confident that if you're reading this book (actually, if you're living in Western society), you are estrogen dominant. It's true—whether you're a woman or a man. Even children are estrogen dominant in this day and age.

This hasn't always been true. It hasn't even been true for the past hundred years. So how did we get here?

Blame xenoestrogens.

HOW ESTROGEN TOOK OVER THE WORLD

After WWII, researchers and industrial corporations were pretty impressed with all the new chemical advancements they were making—especially for agriculture. Through the miracle of science, they cooked up pesticides that protected entire crops, made farms more profitable, and helped keep people fed.[30,31] I'm sure some of them believed they were actually solving world hunger.

From there, they learned to mix and match molecules to create an entire army of synthetic chemicals used in everything from fertilizers to food additives (so food wouldn't spoil), cosmetics and body products (to make them more shelf stable and give them a smooth texture), household cleaners, plastics, and more.

You've probably heard of a few common xenoestrogens, like BPA (Bisphenol A).[30,31] It's found in plastics including water bottles, food containers, and even dental fillings (yikes!). But BPA leaches out of that plastic and enters your body through your water and food. I cringe every time I see someone leave their plastic water bottle in a hot car. That water is swimming with BPA!

Phthalates (pronounced "THAH-lates") are another type of xenoestrogen that pops up everywhere. They're known as "plasticizers," and they make plastic products softer and more flexible.[30,31] They're in vinyl flooring, children's toys, shower curtains, and even shampoo and lotion. (You want plastic in your body lotion, right . . .? Oh wait, *you don't?*)

Then there are parabens (used to make body products feel silky and smooth), dioxins, PCBs, DEHA, and the list goes on and on.

These synthetic molecules are so teeny tiny, they have no problem getting into your body. You eat them, drink them, breathe them in, and even absorb them through your skin. But your body has no idea what these molecules are. It doesn't understand how to process them. So it interprets them as hormones, and they seriously mess up your endocrine system. These particles are fat-soluble, so they can accumulate in your adipose tissue (your body fat). As you read these words, your body could contain xenoestrogens that you were exposed to over 10 years ago. If you lose weight and your fat tissue dissolves, those xenoestrogens get released to circulate through your body again. Now your body finally has the chance to flush them out and detox. You want to be sure your system is as healthy as possible, so they don't stick around and contribute to estrogen dominance.

But they're not safe even after they're detoxed out of your body. Xenoestrogens are not biodegradable. Once they're in the environment, they're there to stay, affecting wildlife, plant life, and future generations of humans.[31]

Back in the 1950s, mad scientists and big corporations didn't stop to research all of this (or if they did, they ignored the results). They were on a roll. They even popularized a quote: "Better living through chemistry!"

I'd like to counter that with another quote: "They were so

preoccupied with whether or not they *could*, that they didn't stop to think if they *should*." (Mine is from *Jurassic Park*!)

And the development of new chemicals hasn't stopped. Millions of new chemicals are created each year, but the EPA is only required to test 20 in the same time frame. You read that right—just 20![32,33] The government doesn't have the funding to keep up. Over in Europe, the European Commission has openly admitted that 99% of chemicals aren't well regulated.[34] It's like we're all part of this ongoing weird science experiment that nobody was consulted on, nobody understood the risks of, and nobody consented to. (I know I sure didn't consent to it!)

Research is slowly trickling in, and it's showing that a lot of these substances can cause cancer.

Well, that explains a lot! We have more cancers now than at any point in history! This isn't random. (I should know. I've had cancer. I was fortunate to have excellent doctors supporting me through that experience, and even more fortunate that the tumor they removed did not metastasize.)

Research is a long, slow process. It can take years to investigate even a few of these chemical synthetics. After scientists finally come to a conclusion on their safety, it can take even longer for legislation to happen that actually bans their use. At this rate, it could be hundreds of years before some of these franken-chemicals are banned! Meanwhile, they've wreaked havoc on our planet and in our bodies in just a few generations.

Do we really need laws to stop them? Yes. It will take

legislation to stop big business from using xenoestrogens. Hey, these chemicals make it cheap and efficient to manufacture a lot of cool stuff! What corporation wouldn't like that?

Consumers have some power, though. People are waking up to the fact that synthetic, processed chemicals are destroying our planet and our health. Pressure on companies to make more natural options is growing, and customers are demanding more transparency around what's in the products they buy. That's excellent news! It's hitting corporations where it hurts: their wallets.

SIGNS AND SYMPTOMS OF ESTROGEN DOMINANCE

How do you know if you're estrogen dominant?

As I mentioned at the opening of this chapter, it's safe to assume that you are. Even if you live as naturally and organically as possible, you're still a resident of Earth. And if you're on the birth control pill or HRT, your endocrine system is in even more of a clusterfrick.

All of the symptoms of low progesterone that I shared in Chapter 3 also indicate estrogen dominance. I don't want to be repetitive and list them all here again, but I will explore three common, serious symptoms that had many of my customers living in fear and misery. (Sadly, that stress may have made their symptoms worse. We'll talk about how to calm stress in Chapter 6.)

Uterine fibroids

These are non-cancerous growths in your uterus. Fibroids are made of smooth muscle and fibrous tissue. They can be tiny or can grow to the size of a grapefruit (or even bigger).

Fibroids are fairly common. Some sources estimate that up to 80% of women have fibroids at some point in their lives (especially during childbearing years; after menopause, they often clear up on their own).

Some women with fibroids are totally symptom-free. Others have to deal with heavy bleeding (for longer than a typical period), cramping, the need to pee a lot, constipation, back pain, and even pregnancy complications or infertility.[35]

If your fibroids are causing pain, your doctor may prescribe the pill, HRT, or surgery. But as with most hormone issues, I recommend using progesterone cream and adjusting your lifestyle. The progesterone can help your body clear out excess estrogen, and fibroids sometimes shrink or stop growing as a result.

Please take note, though: while most fibroids feed off of estrogen, some actually feed off of progesterone. Pay attention to your body and monitor how your fibroids respond to your progesterone cream. If it's not the right product for you, that doesn't mean you should use estrogen instead. If you have fibroids, the last thing you want to do is take estrogen!

Endometriosis

This is a more serious condition. It occurs when uterine

tissue grows outside of the uterus, like around your pelvic organs, on your colon, and even on your lungs.

Endometriosis can cause intense pain, heavy bleeding, and raise your risk of ovarian and breast cancer. Even though it can cause infertility, it is actually possible to get pregnant if you have endometriosis. The condition tends to recede during pregnancy . . . but don't be fooled. It's probably coming back after your normal periods start up again.[36]

Guess what your doctor will probably recommend for this one?

You got it! The pill, HRT, or surgery.

Guess what I say?

Nope, nope, nope! Go with a natural progesterone cream (using similar doses as during early pregnancy) and minimize xenoestrogen exposure. Get regular exercise, so your blood circulates through your body more efficiently. You'll want to adjust your diet, too—check out the suggestions I shared in Chapter 3, or head to Chapter 6 for a clear list of simple ways to get your hormones and health back in balance.

Fibrous breasts

Lumpy, tender, swollen breasts can keep you up at night worrying about cancer, spinning tales of doom in your head about what will happen to your family if you're sick. There's no need to worry about something before you have an official diagnosis, though. You could just have fibrous breasts. They're uncomfortable but not life-threatening. You might find that your breasts feel more tender and lumpier before your period, and then seem to "deflate" after you bleed.[37]

Unless your fibrous breasts are causing you serious trouble (like pain), your doctor will probably recommend that you ignore them.

But again, you can reduce your symptoms (and sometimes even clear up fibrous breasts) by using natural progesterone cream.

DANIEL'S STORY

I was finishing up a conversation with a customer who needed help for uterine fibroids when I noticed a man lurking in the store aisle behind her. He seemed to be examining a lot of products on the shelf very closely, without picking anything up to read the label. I'd seen the behavior before: he was waiting to talk to me.

When I sent the woman away with a red raspberry leaf tincture, the man caught my eye. I smiled, trying to look approachable. Men were sometimes hesitant to speak about their health issues with me.

"Hey there!" I said. "Can I help you find something?"

"Well, I hope so," he said, shuffling forward, hands in his jacket pockets. He was middle-aged with just enough of a belly that spoke of good living without overindulgence. "My doctor says I've got an enlarged prostate."

"Aw, crap!" I said, happy to see him chuckle. "Did he talk to you about it?"

"Yeah, he talked about alpha blockers and surgery. I'm not sure though, I'd really like to see what my natural options are."

"Absolutely, you have plenty of those."

We chatted for the next 15 minutes. His name was Daniel, and his doctor hadn't bothered to look into what caused his prostate issues or asked about concurrent symptoms. Big surprise there! A lot of doctors skip this step (if they consider it a step at all). Digging into the source of a health problem and associated symptoms can take a lot of time, money, and testing.

After all of that, the doctor might still not have an answer. From their point of view, it's more efficient—for both doctor and patient—to just slap a quick solution on the symptom like a band-aid.

Now, I'm not claiming to be some Princess of Prostate Knowledge. I don't have all the answers, and I'm not claiming that all prostate issues are related to estrogen dominance. I'm not a doctor. But I do know that an overload of estrogen in a man's body can lead to an enlarged prostate, cancer, and other issues with the male reproductive system. Maybe that's why I had the courage (or audacity!) to ask Daniel...

"How have things been in the bedroom? Any issues with erections?"

Daniel's eyebrows shot up. He blushed a bit, but said, "Now that you mention it, my sex drive has been pretty low. I never really want it anymore."

I nodded in understanding. I'd seen more and more men—from younger and younger generations—talking about low sex drive. Most of them try to tell themselves it's natural to not want sex very often. But I've been married twice, and I have two sons. I know a thing or two about men! I'm going to come right out and say it: What's between their legs calls the shots! It's a stereotype, but an accurate one. It's not meant to be an insult or something a man should be ashamed of. It's how nature designed men to be.

Ladies, xenoestrogens have been messing with our boys.

According to a 2017 study, sperm counts have dropped by more than 50% since 1973.[38] At the same time, rates of prostate and testicular cancers have tripled. Reproductive abnormalities like undescended testicles have gotten more and more common in Europe and the United States.

Research also shows that when pregnant women are exposed to widespread chemicals, their baby boys have smaller penises and even feminized genitals. Gwynne Lyons, a former government advisor on the health effects of chemicals, summed it up when she said, "This research shows that the basic male tool kit is under threat."[39]

It's no coincidence that transgenderism is on the rise in younger generations. They've been exposed to high levels of xenoestrogens, aka "gender benders," since they were in the womb. Their parents were exposed for most of their lives, too.

As he opened up about his lack of libido, Daniel admitted

with defeat, "I figured a lower sex drive is just part of getting older."

"Well, yes and no," I said. "It's natural for your sex drive to decrease a bit, but you're not old enough to lose your libido altogether! You've probably been exposed to too much estrogen."

He laughed. "My wife hates when I make that joke!"

I laughed too, and then explained the xenoestrogen situation to Daniel.

"So I *really was* exposed to too much estrogen!"

"You really were! I'm going to put you on some topical progesterone cream and some nutrients for prostate health. It may help reduce the size of your prostate, and it'll serve as a precursor for your body to make more testosterone."

A few months later, Daniel came back to see me, a big smile on his face. He shook my hand and said his prostate was shrinking, and he'd been having sex with his wife more often. His doctor (and his wife) didn't know where the changes were coming from . . . but they weren't complaining!

XENOESTROGENS ARE CHANGING OUR WILDLIFE

Estrogen dominance is not your fault.

Xenoestrogens are so prevalent in our environment that it's impossible to avoid them. Even if you only buy organic non-GMO food; even if you clean your home with pure vinegar and castile soap; even if you only use the most natural, crunchy-granola, fragrance-free makeup brands . . .

xenoestrogens are in your water, in your carpets, in the upholstery and dashboard of your car, and in the air of the store you strolled through to pick up your niece's birthday present.

Even wildlife can't escape these agents of chaos!

In Florida, biologists discovered something strange going on with the alligators in Lake Apopka. To understand what was happening, they looked at the history of the area. They found that in 1980, a toxic spill dumped huge amounts of a pesticide similar to DDT into the lake. Five years later, 90% of the alligators had disappeared. Of the remaining 10%, most were incapable of reproducing or had no urge to mate. The males were born with penises that were not only 75% shorter than the average length but were also deformed. Their testosterone levels were so low that they resembled females.

Speaking of the females, they had abnormal ovaries and follicles, which biologists described as "burned out."[40,41]

No alligators were getting it on in Lake Apopka.

In Canada, fish swimming in water polluted by a pulp mill were either late to sexually mature or developed as hermaphrodites.[31]

Fish in the UK showed similar traits. Male fish downstream from sewage treatment plants changed their sex as a result of estrogen chemicals that were still in the sewage waste.[42]

These events aren't random. They're not a sign that life is evolving to be less "binary" with fewer clear lines between males and females. Nature designed us male and female to keep the species reproducing—and reproduction is one of Mama Nature's Big Objectives. She doesn't compromise on that. She doesn't create species that don't want to (or can't) mate and reproduce. These chemicals cause changes to human and animal DNA that result in physical reproductive abnormalities.

And since the changes happen in the DNA, they can be passed on to our offspring.

AN UNPRECEDENTED PROBLEM IN HUMAN HISTORY

We're dealing with a completely unprecedented situation in history. Our foremothers wouldn't know what to do in our shoes. They lived in a world that wasn't flooded with chemicals. So we're trying to figure out the problem and find solutions at the same time.

If you talk to your doctor, she won't know what to do other than treat your symptoms. She may want to put you on birth control pills or HRT—without understanding that all those synthetic hormones and estrogen contributed to the issue in the first place, and more will only make the issue worse.

She might even resort to procedures like ablation, D&C, or hysterectomy.

If at all possible, I highly urge you to avoid these procedures.

Ablation is usually recommended for women who have uncontrollable bleeding. In this procedure, the doctor essentially scorches the inside of your uterus, your endometrium. Picture the inside of a cave that's been burned with a flamethrower. The walls are dry and scorched black.

Ablation prevents your uterine lining from growing. That may sound great if you're bleeding so heavily that you can't leave the house . . . but ablation also stops your uterus and vagina's natural self-cleaning process.

Your lady bits are pretty cool. They clean themselves, creating mucus that naturally flows from your uterus, cervix, and vaginal walls. It's thick, sticky, and liquid enough that it basically rinses you out from within. It also keeps your vaginal microbiome balanced. Without that natural cleaning, there's nothing to keep out unhealthy bacteria. Vaginosis makes itself right at home.

As for hysterectomy, if you're in your childbearing years, it sends your body into early menopause. Hysterectomy completely removes your body's ability to naturally produce its own estrogen and progesterone. Even if your doctor leaves your ovaries intact, they'll likely stop producing hormones in a few years.

Is this all starting to sound stressful?

Don't worry, there's no need to stress! (Especially because stress can make hormone issues worse.)

So what should you do? I've got your complete map for hormone balance in Chapter 6.

Before I lay out all of your options, I want to touch on another set of diseases that are often related to endocrine disorders: autoimmune issues.

5

HORMONES & AUTOIMMUNE DISEASE

"Health is a state of complete mental, social and physical well-being, not merely the absence of disease or infirmity."

— WORLD HEALTH ORGANIZATION, 1948

I like to compare the immune system to a nation's construction crews and military.

Why construction crews? A nation is made of roads, buildings, cities, and a ton of infrastructure that has the tendency to break down if it's not regularly repaired. Your immune system does that for your body. It's constantly rebuilding you after you get injured, or simply after the everyday wear and tear of living your life.

Why the military? Because a nation also has to fight off invaders. Your immune system does that beautifully.

It's engaged in both of these actions all the time. We're talking 24 hours a day, 7 days a week, 365 days a year. It's even hard at work while you sleep. (In fact, sleep is essential for your immune system to function. When you're sleeping, that's when the "night crew" comes on shift—a whole little army of cells that repair inflammation and polish you up, so you feel refreshed the next day. If you've ever gone to bed with a headache and woken up feeling better, that's why.)

If the "military" side of your immune system encounters a brand new enemy—a pathogen or something it's never seen before—it works overtime to learn, evolve, and meet the new threat.

Your immune system has a big job. So when it's not working as it should, it can spell serious trouble for your health and happiness.

An autoimmune issue arises when your body's immune system gets confused and starts attacking healthy organs, tissues, or other cells. It's like a nation's soldiers turning against the citizens because they simply can't tell friend from foe anymore. The soldiers themselves aren't bad. They've just been given confusing orders.

Of course, if your immune system is attacking your body, a host of debilitating symptoms and conditions can arise. Autoimmune issues are no picnic. Trust me—I've been there. (I'll share my story at the end of this chapter.)

Women, unfortunately, are four times more likely to

develop autoimmune diseases than men.[43] Researchers aren't 100% sure why. They have a bunch of educated guesses like:

- Our hormones fluctuate a lot throughout our lives, and much of our health depends on maintaining a delicate balance.
- Our microbiomes are different from men's.
- Maybe when we get pregnant, tiny amounts of fetal cells somehow manage to circulate through our body, alerting our immune system of foreign invaders. (It's called "microchimerism," and it's kind of similar to what happens when the immune system attacks a transplanted organ.)
- Environmental factors. (This is what scientists say when they think something external caused the problem, but they have no idea what.)

Whatever the reasons, we're more vulnerable to autoimmune problems.

It's not easy to list symptoms of autoimmune disorders, because there are so many different types of disorders affecting different organs or tissues. But a few examples include rheumatoid arthritis (which affects your joints), multiple sclerosis (affecting your brain, spinal cord, and optic nerves, leading to system-wide dysfunction), lupus (affecting a wide variety of tissues throughout your body), and type 1 diabetes (affecting insulin-producing cells). Even inflammatory bowel disease is an autoimmune disorder (affecting your digestive tract).

HORMONES AND YOUR IMMUNE SYSTEM

It really gets my goat when doctors don't try to get at the root of what's causing an autoimmune disorder. Sometimes it seems like they'll try anything to treat the condition . . . anything *except* understanding and healing its source! I won't tell you that I fully understand the source of every autoimmune disorder. I don't have a medical degree.

But I do understand how influential hormones are. There's a saying I've shared with many of my customers and clients: *We are walking hormones.* These little messengers are like pieces of software code swimming throughout your body. The code tells your organs and physiological systems what to do. If the code gets corrupted or malware is introduced, your entire body is affected.

I've seen hundreds of autoimmune issues clear up when underlying hormonal imbalances are addressed. (I'm including my own autoimmune issues here. Doctors had no clue what was causing my condition! It turned out to be hormone-related.)

Let's start by talking about the culprit behind most of the problems we've talked about in this book . . .

Estrogen

It's not easy to sum up estrogen's relationship to your

immune response. But in general, estrogen has an activating effect on your immune system.

High levels of estrogen can stimulate the production of your T-cells (which destroy cancerous cells) and B-cells (which create antibodies that fight pathogens and invaders).[44] That's fine if you're actually sick. But if you're not, all those immune cells become confused soldiers, looking for something to attack. Sometimes they decide to attack healthy cells.

Your estrogen can also stimulate the excess production of pro-inflammatory cytokines, which activate your inflammation response.[45] Again, that's fine if you're sick. "Pro-inflammatory" may sound scary, but your body actually uses inflammation to fight infection and repair damage. So your pro-inflammatory cytokines are usually working in your favor.

That changes if there are too many of them constantly floating around. Now your inflammation response is going wild!

Too much estrogen can also affect your gut, leading to "leaky gut" that allows estrogen to be reabsorbed *from* your gut, *back into* your bloodstream.[46] Talk about a shitty estrogen effect! No, thank you! That can lead to a whole other set of immune disorders, including IBS.

Estrogen can even alter genes that control your immune regulation, meaning your genetic code has been rewritten to include an immune disorder.[44]

Doctors might be scratching their heads about why women are more vulnerable to immune disorders . . . but I don't feel quite so confused. Considering how awash our lives are in xenoestrogens, it's a wonder that more people aren't walking around with autoimmunity. There's even evidence that women who have taken the pill or HRT for many years have a higher incidence of rheumatoid arthritis and lupus.[47]

After menopause, when your progesterone levels sink to practically nothing, you're even more vulnerable to estrogen-influenced autoimmunity.

Progesterone

Because low progesterone occurs hand in hand with high estrogen, it's associated with all the problems I mentioned earlier, under the "estrogen" section. You want to keep your progesterone levels healthy, so it can balance out the estrogen.

Thyroid

I could write a whole book on thyroid issues! (And I have one planned . . . Check my website at HealthyLivingByLiz.com to see if it's published by the time you're reading this!) As a reminder, your thyroid affects your metabolism, growth, and calcium levels. That's why it plays a significant role in your weight and bone density.

If your immune system attacks your thyroid, you can develop Hashimoto's thyroiditis—hypothyroidism. You'll gain weight with this condition because it slows down your metabolism. Your body can't process calories at a healthy rate. You'll gain weight no matter how healthy your diet is (sometimes up to 30 pounds!). Most of this weight is due to your body holding onto excess water and salt.[48,49]

But your immune system can also create antibodies that overstimulate your thyroid, leading to Grave's disease—hyperthyroidism. With this condition, you'll lose weight. That may not seem like a big deal at first (you might even welcome it!), but it means your body isn't using energy effectively. You may feel hungrier, but your body won't hold onto the food you're giving it, leading to malnutrition. Eventually, the body resorts to breaking down its own tissues (and even bone) to get the energy it needs.[48,49]

Both conditions are also marked by mood swings that leave you feeling helpless to control your emotions.

While thyroid issues are complicated and can stem from different causes, estrogen dominance can be a source of the problem.[50]

In fact, symptoms of hypothyroidism—like fatigue, weight gain, and feeling cold all the time—can look a lot like symptoms of estrogen dominance. If you have these symptoms, your doctor might test you for hypothyroidism, only to be confused when the test comes back negative. She won't understand the term "estrogen dominance" and she won't know how to test for the condition.

I suggest using natural progesterone cream. If your symptoms are estrogen-related, the cream will help. If they're thyroid-related, it still won't hurt!

Cortisol

Earlier in this book, I explained why it's important to have healthy levels of stress hormones. You want your stress response to get activated by... well... *stress*! It has to keep you safe in the face of danger. That's why it elevates your heart rate, makes you breathe faster, gives you a rush of energy, dilates your blood vessels, and even widens your pupils so you can take in more light. All of these physical responses help you get away from that angry bear (or from your boss on a rampage)!

When your stress hormones, including cortisol, are too high or too low, everything starts to tip out of balance—even your immune system. Cortisol's relationship to autoimmunity is complicated, but I'll give you an overview.

The basic thing to understand is that cortisol has anti-inflammatory effects that suppress the immune system.[51] After all, if you're fighting a bear, your body is facing a more immediate threat than the common cold. Cortisol directs your resources toward the more immediate danger.

These anti-inflammatory effects are why cortisol-based steroid medications are often prescribed for skin allergies, like hives. In an allergy, your immune system decides a seemingly innocent substance is dangerous. Your immune system shouts, "Danger, Will Robinson!" It sends an army of immune cells that create inflammation to heal you (not understanding that it's actually causing damage).

Cortisol cream reduces the number of your immune cells.[52] The small army of immune cells that do show up to the fight is less active, sluggishly trying to fend off threats. That gives your irritated skin time to actually heal. And that's how cortisol creams work to soothe dermatitis and skin allergies.[52]

So it makes sense that if you have an autoimmune disorder, short periods of high cortisol (lasting a few weeks or so) can actually reduce your symptoms for a while.

But prolonged periods of high cortisol are a different story. If stress or anxiety becomes chronic, your cortisol reserves get depleted. Now, after the stress subsides, you're actually dealing with *low cortisol*.[53]

As we've touched on, chronically low levels of cortisol are no good.

The cortisol isn't around to suppress the immune response, so your immune system gets overactive. Let's return to the metaphor of your immune system being like an army. When your cortisol is too low, it's like the drill sergeant didn't show up to make sure all the soldiers went "lights out" at bedtime. Now the soldiers are awake and gunning for a fight! They'll beat up anybody who crosses their path . . . even your healthy tissues!

If your cortisol levels are chronically low, there are a few things you can do. Find ways to calm any chronic stress or anxiety that you struggle with. (You'll find tips in Chapter 6.) At the same time, take steps to stimulate your adrenal glands. I know, it might sound counterintuitive to stimulate your adrenals if you have chronic stress! But you want to get a healthy cortisol level flowing through your system. Make sure to get regular exercise (if your energy is low, start small;

even gentle movement is better than no movement), and use natural progesterone cream.

Progesterone is the precursor to cortisol.

If your estrogen is high and your progesterone is low, then your body doesn't have the main ingredient to make cortisol. Take care of your progesterone, and it will take care of you.

Testosterone

Like the other hormones I've talked about in this chapter, testosterone's relationship to immune health doesn't always seem straightforward. It's not as simple as "low testosterone leads to autoimmunity." That said, I'm going to generalize once again and say that while estrogen tends to activate the immune response, testosterone tends to suppress it.

Testosterone has anti-inflammatory effects that help regulate a man's immune response, stopping it from working overtime.[54] So if his testosterone is low, his immune system might just stay on high alert, looking for unhealthy cells or invaders to destroy . . . and, when it doesn't find them, turning on healthy tissues. That's why in men, low testosterone can lead to autoimmunity.

Low testosterone is linked to serious problems even when autoimmunity isn't part of the picture. One study on hospital patients suffering from sepsis found that 70% of male patients died from the condition, compared to 25% of female patients who died. All of the men who died had low levels of testosterone.[55]

High testosterone isn't necessarily better, though. In a

study, men with high testosterone received a flu vaccine, but they didn't produce as many antibodies in response to the shot as women and men with lower levels of the hormone.[56] An overload of testosterone can even affect a man's immune system on the genetic level.[56]

This is a very basic overview of testosterone's effect on autoimmunity. There's a lot of confusing, conflicting information out there. The basic tenet holds true: both men and women need balanced, healthy testosterone to prevent autoimmune issues. And progesterone is the precursor to testosterone. It's the great balancer! That's why even men can benefit from using natural progesterone cream.

GENETICS AND AUTOIMMUNE ISSUES

Are you thinking, *"Liz, you've mentioned autoimmune diseases like multiple sclerosis, rheumatoid arthritis, and Hashimoto's. But these are genetic diseases. There's nothing I can do about an autoimmune disease in my genes!"*

You're right—a lot of autoimmune disorders are genetic. The program for the disease is written in your genes, and as you get older and go about your life, those genes might get triggered and turn on. But that doesn't mean you're doomed. A genetic predisposition for a disease isn't necessarily a ticking time bomb.

Your lifestyle plays a huge role in your health, including how some of your genes express themselves.

Have you ever heard stories of identical twins who were

separated at birth and raised in completely different lifestyles? One was raised eating meat and potatoes followed by a slice of apple pie. The other grew up eating plenty of green veggies and grilled chicken with Greek yogurt and berries for dessert. One grew up playing video games all day, while the other got outside regularly and developed a healthy habit of exercise. And when they grow up, one develops rheumatoid arthritis, while the other continues happily running and climbing stairs without joint pain for years.

A lifestyle that stresses your immune system is more likely to trigger a latent autoimmune disorder in your genes.

Doctors won't often talk about the role of diet and exercise in autoimmune disorders. Why? I'll explain by quoting one of my own doctors. Years ago, I was told my liver enzymes were out of balance. (That's not an autoimmune issue, but my interaction with my doctor explains a lot about the medical mindset.) My doctor wanted to put me on some new miracle drug, but I asked for a grace period of three months.

"I want to try addressing this with diet and nutrition."

"Liz, that stuff doesn't work," he said, rolling his eyes.

"Give me three months," I said again.

At which he shrugged and said, "Okay, three months."

I buried my head in my books and put myself on a new diet and supplement regimen. After three months, my doctor's jaw literally dropped when he saw my test results.

"What did you do?" he asked. "Your levels are back to normal!"

I laughed. "Oh no, I'm not telling!" I joked. "My stuff doesn't work, remember? The change must be a miracle!"

He laughed, too, but was serious when he explained, "Liz, you have to understand, I wasn't taught this stuff. Yes, I went through years of medical school, and I have an M.D., but we weren't taught about nutrition. We were led to believe it doesn't play a very significant role. So when you said you could heal yourself with nutrition, I doubted you. And when I see results like yours, I'm just blown away. I have no frame of reference for understanding it. You have a completely different knowledge base than I can draw from."

I almost felt sorry for him. He was a good man and he truly wanted to help his patients. But even though he'd gone through *all that schooling*, his education had left him with significant knowledge gaps that often prevented him from offering people the most natural, noninvasive solutions. The pharmaceutical companies constantly inundating him with brochures about new drugs weren't helping him out, either.

So I explained my liver-enzyme healing protocol and watched him take notes.

MY ROAD TO HELL AND BACK

If you're struggling with autoimmunity, my heart goes out to you. Autoimmunity can take many different shapes, and none of them are a picnic. I speak from experience. In my life, I've dealt with cancer, liver issues, and an autoimmune disease called Charcot-Marie-Tooth (CMT). CMT is an inherited genetic disease that attacks nerve cells. There is no known cure, and an advanced case can be life-altering.

But the worst health struggle I've ever dealt with was a different autoimmune issue altogether.

The story starts way back in 2008 when the financial crisis was in full swing. Like a million other people, I lost everything: my job, car, home, retirement, and even a seven-year relationship I had come to cherish and rely on. In a very short time, the beautiful life I had built for myself collapsed. I felt like I was left with nothing. After that, my life became a whirlwind of stress. It remained that way for a long, long, awfully long time.

Fast-forward to November of 2010, and I had been living in constant stress for two years. The day after Thanksgiving, I woke up covered in raised, red, itchy, painful bumps. I was terrified! I had no idea what was happening! I thought, "Oh crap . . . what did I eat last night to bring up a reaction like this?" But I couldn't think of anything out of the ordinary. I'd had all of my family's classic dishes, and it was all food that I had eaten many times. Maybe something foreign had gotten into one of the dishes? Or one of the food companies I bought from had started using a different processing method, or new sources of ingredients?

I had no idea. I took care of myself as well as I could. But after a week, the bumps were still there.

Well, time to get back into my favorite pastime: research!

I dug through all of my most reliable books and combed the internet. I found dozens of possible explanations ... but not one that actually felt on target. At my wits' end, I finally broke down and went to an allergist. That appointment changed my life.

The allergist diagnosed me with chronic idiopathic urticaria—basically, chronic hives with no known cause. So: mystery hives. Great. I could have told the doctor that!

Fast-forward again to 2012. My mystery hives were still going strong (yup, I'd had them every day for a full two years!), and I was once again the owner of a vitamin shop. I had nurtured a reputation as a local natural health guru... but here I was, chronically covered in painful, itchy welts! I looked like a monster. It wasn't exactly reassuring for my customers, who wanted to trust that I knew a lot about natural healing. And up until this point, I had thought I did!

My research rabbit hole continued, reaching all the way to China and back. I tried to zero in on what I should or shouldn't eat. I checked my clothing, my bedding, and all the detergents and cleaners in my house. I looked into my soap, lotion, shampoos, and makeup. I even looked at local industries around my house. Maybe some company was dumping chemicals in the soil or water supply?

I couldn't find *anything*.

By now, you probably know I'm the type of person who avoids pharmaceutical drugs at all costs. But this was an emergency situation, and I didn't know what else to do. I tried different medications from my doctor, including prednisone (a corticosteroid) and any kind of allergy meds that wouldn't put me to sleep. I also had to take a stomach antacid. Having to take all these pills was devastating. But I was miserable. *I would have tried literally anything.* If I had thought heroin would make these painful hives go away, I would have been shooting up every night!

Even with all the meds, the hives still came daily. Some mornings I would wake up clear (but they would always pop up later!), and others I would wake up scratching. And this itch wasn't your average mosquito bite, where you can scratch and bleed and get a scab. Oh no, this went deep into my skin. *It hurt all over.* One time, the hives even broke out in my eyes. Yup—I got hives on my eyeballs. They turned bloodred and swelled shut. That was fun.

This autoimmune issue even affected my hearing. I became deaf in one ear, and hearing aids couldn't do anything for the type of hearing loss I had.

Every day, whether I woke up with hives or not, they'd definitely start popping up around nine o'clock in the evening. It was like clockwork, so predictable that I started calling my condition "Vampire's Disease." My roommate could sit next to me on the couch and watch the hives appear before her eyes. If I went out to eat with friends, I had to make sure I was home in time for my nightly transformation into a monster. Otherwise, I'd feel the hives coming on during the main course. I'd have to call for a doggie bag and get out of there fast! I would have been a great addition to

P.T. Barnum's sideshow—the lady who transforms into a polka-dotted monster every night!

At bedtime, I would do my best to calm down and relax. Sometimes it worked, others . . . not so much. The pain and itching would often wake me up in the middle of the night. Even the sheets touching my skin could be overwhelming. Now sleeplessness compounded my stress. I'm sure my lack of sleep made the hives worse.

All this time, my doctor was helping me try to find an answer. He was a great ally and would pull any blood work I asked for. Eventually, he tossed up his hands and said, "Liz, this is easily one of the worst cases I've ever seen. I'd like to put you on a regimen of chemo and see if that helps."

That's when I knew that, despite his good intentions, he was at a complete loss for how to help me. Chemotherapy? For hives?

I said, "Nope. Not doing that."

With no answers from medical science or in my research, I started contemplating suicide. At this point, the Hives from Hell had been plaguing me every day for four years. My life had become near-constant misery. I just wanted it to end. I couldn't stop thinking of ways to do it, and I came up with some doozies! My sons were both grown, so they didn't need me as much as they had when they were younger. I started trying to prepare them for my suicide. I know that sounds hideous, but I had nowhere to turn, and I couldn't keep living in such pain. I would slip half-joking statements into our conversations like, "This is no way to live my life," but I don't think either of them ever took me seriously.

One day, four years into this nightmare, I had a very disturbing phone call from a business partner. I won't go into details, but I will say that it sent my stress through the roof. At this time, I was about a year and a half into menopause. I'd never had any of the dreaded symptoms, like hot flashes or night sweats, but I hadn't bled for 18 months so I knew I was probably through the change.

Even so, I hung up that phone, and within two hours I was bleeding. This wasn't any light spotting, either. This was a full-on period. I was flabbergasted. What was going on? Was it even possible to have a period after menopause? At first, I was very concerned...

However, my fears quickly subsided.

Because for the full week that I was bleeding, *my hives went away.*

I couldn't believe it! I was hive-free! I'd been fighting these monster hives every day for four years with no reprieve. Now, all of a sudden, they were gone. That week reminded me of what life could be like without constant itching and pain.

But once the bleeding stopped, guess what? The hives came roaring back with a vengeance—like they wanted to punish me for getting a short break.

This experience got me thinking about hives in a whole new way. They had stopped during my period. Could they possibly be hormone-related? I got out my research books and read every hormone study I could find. I realized that the stressful call from my business partner had really shaken up my hormones, starting my period, and that my hormones had probably been unbalanced all this time. I immediately got on natural progesterone cream, following the instructions on the label religiously and applying it every night before bed.

About three months of being on the progesterone cream, I woke up one morning . . . and there were no hives. I crossed my fingers and waited for their usual appearance at nine o'clock. They didn't show. They didn't show up that night or the next morning, either.

By this point, I was both excited and scared. I loved being hive-free! But I was terrified that they would come back. That fear stayed with me for two weeks. I walked on eggshells every minute of those 14 days, worried I would eat the wrong thing or do something to bring back my torture. But the torture didn't come back. Eventually, I had to tell myself, "C'mon, Liz, you're stressing out about feeling healthy? That's a little overboard, don't you think?" I got serious about trying to manage my stress.

To this day, I'm happily hive-free. Of course, I didn't end my life. I get to enjoy more time with my sons and their families. Not a day goes by that I don't feel grateful for my health and my life.

As time passed, I thought more about my harrowing hives ordeal. I realized that my hormonal menopause issues, combined with the constant stress I'd been living with since

2008, had probably triggered the hives. Stress is the killer of everything, and I can't "stress that" enough. Chronic stress sends all of your hormones haywire. And I'll say it again: *You are a walking hormone.* An imbalance of one hormone can affect your entire system. It can manifest symptoms you'd never expect, and which baffle your doctors. When your hormones aren't healthy, *you* aren't healthy. Take care of your hormones, and they will take care of you.

I took before and after pictures of my hives journey. Nothing brings home the magic of this transformation like seeing the red bumpy blotches of my hive-covered hide, compared with my clear, healthy skin after I started using progesterone cream again.

See the pictures by scanning the QR code and visiting my website.

HORMONE BALANCE MADE SIMPLE

"Those who think they have no time for healthy eating will soon have to find time for illness."

— EDWARD STANLEY

This chapter is your step-by-step guide for balancing your hormones naturally! You'll learn how to minimize your exposure to xenoestrogens, eat for hormone health, manage stress, make your own cleaning products (toxin-free!), exercise more regularly, get enough healthy sleep to keep your endocrine system happy, and more.

There's a lot of information in this chapter, but there's no need to get overwhelmed or stressed out trying to overhaul your entire life. You don't have to implement every single aspect of this plan. The idea is to minimize stress—not freak out even more about all the healthy stuff you're not doing!

That said, I encourage you to do your best, especially if you're:

- Struggling to get pregnant.
- Going through a difficult menopause.
- Not having periods.
- Having dangerously heavy periods.
- Dealing with fibroids.
- Sick with autoimmune issues.
- Trying to get off of the birth control pill or HRT.
- Trying to cope with other hormone-related issues that are wreaking havoc on your life.

I'm not telling you to ignore your doctor. I'm saying you have the power to take your health into your own hands. I want your doctor to be surprised and thrilled by how well you're doing!

Of course, my first bit of advice is almost always going to be to use natural progesterone cream. You can also try some of the progesterone support herbs I mentioned in Chapter 3. In addition to all that goodness, let's get into key lifestyle changes that can transform your health. These recommendations hold true for women, men, and children.

DIET

You are what you eat! Can you put water in the gas tank and expect the car to run? Your body can't create a recipe for balanced hormones if it doesn't have all of the ingredients.

I'll share specific foods to put on your plate and others you should avoid, but first I want to talk about eating habits and weight in general. Because it's true that your hormones influence your weight. If you're overweight and your hormones are unbalanced, it can trap you in an unhealthy cycle that keeps your hormones confused and makes it feel impossible to lose weight and keep it off.

The connection between weight gain and hormones

Let's start with the hormone insulin. A lot of people are familiar with this little guy. Insulin allows your cells to process sugar (glucose) for energy, and it keeps your blood sugar regulated. But when your pancreas doesn't produce enough insulin—maybe because you eat too many carbs or sweets, and that dietary sugar is always circulating in your blood (your body changes carbs into glucose)—you'll develop insulin resistance. That leads to weight gain and, in some cases, diabetes.[57,58]

Then there's our good friend leptin, which is made by your body fat. Your insulin tells your fat to send leptin messengers to your brain. Once there, leptin says, "Hey, Brain, we've got enough energy stored in our body fat. We don't need to eat any more right now!" And that's why you don't feel hungry all the time . . . or why you *shouldn't* feel hungry all the time. If your insulin is unbalanced or if you're fat, your body might have higher levels of leptin, but your brain might be desensitized to it. That can make it feel like you need to eat more and more to produce enough leptin to actually feel full.[57,58]

Leptin and insulin help regulate one another.

Unbalanced cortisol (everyone's favorite stress hormone) can make you gain weight, too.[57,58] During an acute stress response, you might actually lose weight. That's because cortisol is trying to save you from a pack of hyenas or tight deadlines at work. It's pulling reserves of energy from your fat, surging strength through your body so you can get to safety. During that time, it suppresses appetite. Who has time to eat when hyenas are attacking? But after the danger passes, you'll probably feel pretty hungry. You have to replenish your lost energy reserves.

But if your cortisol levels are constantly too high, then a shift happens. Now your body responds by feeling hungry more often. You're obviously surrounded by hyenas all the time and need as much energy as possible to escape at a moment's notice.

Of course, HGH affects your weight, too. That's the hormone that regulates your metabolism and growth. It keeps your metabolism going strong while you're growing because you need a lot of energy from food to build bones and muscles. But when HGH gets depleted or unbalanced, your metabolism slows down. Now you gain weight more easily.

And what about your sex hormones, estrogen, progesterone, and testosterone? What kind of an impact do they have on your weight?

A big one!

Estrogen tells a woman's body to collect fat around the hips, butt, and thighs. It's also stored in your body fat.[57,58] So the more fat you have, the more estrogen you have. I've said it before, and I'll say it again: We're told that postmenopausal women are dealing with estrogen shortages. But a fat older woman has more estrogen in her body than a thin younger woman. Keep your estrogen and progesterone balanced to help maintain a healthy weight.

In men, low testosterone is associated with high body fat and low muscle mass.[57,58] Men with a lot of muscle burn calories more efficiently than men with a lot of fat. It might seem unfair, but this means muscled men can eat more without getting fat. Their muscles need all of that food to convert into energy! But if his testosterone is low, he's going to have trouble building muscles. Now all that food turns into fat. Low testosterone is also associated with insulin resistance . . . and we've already discussed what happens to your weight when that happens!

In my decades of work at vitamin and supplement stores, I've talked to hundreds of people who said their weight was due to hormonal issues. Yet they were constantly trying to approach weight loss with diet and exercise. Those are important, for sure . . . but it never occurred to a lot of people that they could reach a healthier weight by balancing their hormones.

On the other hand, not eating enough of the right types of food can cause a body weight that's way too low. That's what happened to Josie, whose story you read in Chapter 3. She believed she was eating a healthy diet. But she wasn't giving her body the right ingredients to build a healthy endocrine system, have periods, and make a baby. She needed more healthy cholesterol so her body could create estrogen and progesterone.

Types of foods to avoid

Let's get into the nitty-gritty! Here's a list of foods to cross off your shopping list. One or two servings of this stuff won't hurt, but if eating them becomes a habit, they'll change your hormones for the worse.

- **Factory-raised red meat:** Red meat is high in saturated fat, which can increase estrogen levels.[59] That said, I actually like organic, grass-fed red meat. The factory-raised animals (along with being treated miserably) are usually pumped full of hormones to make them fat and meaty. You don't need to eat these hormones.
- **Soy:** Soy contains phytoestrogens, which can mimic estrogen and disrupt hormone balance.[60] And remember: women in Asian countries stay slim and never have hot flashes because they eat soy . . . but they're eating a different kind of soy

than is available in the United States and most Western countries.

- **Dairy:** Cow milk is for calves, and most dairy products contain synthetic hormones. Like animals raised in factories for their meat, factory dairy cows are put on hormones, so their udders stay full of milk.
- **Caffeine:** A daily coffee habit can increase cortisol levels, leading to weight gain and other health issues.[61]
- **Processed foods:** These so-called "foods" include fast food, bagged chips, plastic-wrapped cakes, breakfast cereals, processed meats like bacon, and more. They're often high in sugar, salt, and unhealthy fats, which can disrupt your hormones.
- **Alcohol:** Every now and then, your local news might feature a study that shows a few health benefits of alcohol and encourages you to "have a glass of red wine tonight." I hope that sets off your bullshit detector! Alcohol is not good for your body, period. When it comes to your hormones, alcohol can raise your estrogen, lower testosterone, screw with your thyroid, lead to insulin resistance, disrupt your sleep-wake cycle, interfere with your adrenals and cortisol levels, and more.[62] If you want the healthy polyphenols and resveratrol in red wine, get them from

antioxidant-rich fruits and veggies. (Just eat the grapes!)

Types of foods to eat

I can't encourage you enough to eat more plants!

Plants are chock-full of the good stuff that gives your body all the ingredients for healthy hormones, including vitamins, minerals, antioxidants, and fiber. They can even reduce the risk of serious diseases like breast cancer and endometriosis. You'll also find some healthy proteins on this list (and in the "What's on the menu?" section below), but the biggest section of your plate should be reserved for plants.

Protein contains protein. Plants contain nutrients.

- **Cruciferous veggies:** Broccoli, cauliflower, kale, and other cruciferous vegetables contain I3C, which makes your estrogen receptors less . . . well, less *receptive*.[63] They also protect you from estrogen-based DNA damage.
- **A rainbow of other veggies:** A good rule of thumb is to eat the rainbow (and I'm not talking about colorful little candies!). Different colored veggies contain different nutrients and antioxidants, all of which are important for your endocrine system.
- **Good fats:** Healthy fats such as avocados, nuts, and olive oil contain polyunsaturated fats, like omega-3 fatty acid, which supports progesterone.[64]

- **Quality protein:** Lean sources of protein such as chicken, fish, salmon, and tofu can boost your progesterone, and regulate insulin and cortisol. I also like organic, grass-fed red meat.[65]
- **Flaxseeds and oil:** Along with being rich in healthy fatty acids, flaxseeds contain lignans, which can help balance estrogen levels.[66]
- **Whole fruit:** Whole fruit is a great source of fiber and antioxidants, but remember, fruit is still mostly sugar. Don't go fruitarian and eat nothing but fruit. (And fruit juice doesn't have the same benefits. It only gives you the sugar and some of the nutrients from fruit while stripping out the fiber.)
- **Healthy carbs:** Whole grains such as quinoa and brown rice are high in fiber, which helps regulate insulin.[67]
- **Herbs and spices:** Herbs and spices such as turmeric, cinnamon, and ginger can help reduce inflammation and support hormone balance.

A note about gut health

I've mentioned the importance of gut health a few times. Now I'd like to explain it a little more thoroughly (although this is still a very quick overview of the topic).

If I could talk to a 20-year-old me, I might give her a warning: "Get ready to learn more about intestines and poop than you ever thought you'd know! There's *a lot of research* on this topic in your future!" At one of my vitamin stores, I even earned the playful nickname "The Poop Queen" because I helped so many people heal their guts and have healthier bowel movements!

Your gut microbiome sounds gross when you're first learning about it. It's a complex ecosystem of bacteria, viruses, fungi, and other little critters that live in your intestines. This little community works together to keep your digestion healthy and ensures your body actually gets access to the nutrients you eat. Your small intestine is in charge of this (not, as some people think, your stomach). It absorbs the nutrients and distributes them into your bloodstream. Your gut is also a big player when it comes to your metabolism and immune response.

It plays a huge role in your hormone health, too. Your gut is involved in the production of hormones, how your body metabolizes hormones, and the elimination of hormones.[68,69]

If your gut isn't healthy, you can develop IBS (Irritable Bowel Syndrome), Crohn's disease, SIBO (small intestine bacterial overgrowth), candida and yeast infections (which can even show up in your mouth, where it's called oral thrush), food sensitivities, gas, bloating, poor nutrient absorption, and even autoimmune issues.[68,69]

Leaky gut is another common problem. That's what happens when your gut lining becomes thin and more permeable than it should be.[68,69] Now it's not only nutrients being absorbed into your bloodstream, but toxins that your body is trying to eliminate. One of these is excess estrogen. Let's say your body manages to identify an army of xenoestrogens running wild and sabotaging your health, and it decides to get rid of them. Excellent! Glad to see your body recognizing the problem! It sends the army of xenoestrogens to your gut . . . which then sends them right back into your bloodstream. Now that army is right back to its old shenanigans, and it's compounding the effects of new estrogen, xenoestrogens, and synthetic hormones that are introduced into your system.

Other things that permeate your leaky gut lining? Larger protein molecules, which don't belong in your bloodstream and which your immune system targets like foreign invaders. Cue autoimmune issues![68,69]

Women on the birth control pill or HRT are at a higher risk for gut issues.[70]

You can't heal your hormones without healing your gut. And you heal your gut with food and supplements. Make sure to eat plenty of fiber-rich and fermented foods (like kimchi, sauerkraut, and kombucha). Fermented foods contain pre- and probiotics that help populate your gut microbiome with the good guys. If you take the birth control pill or HRT, or if you're trying to stop, you've got to make friends with probiotics.

Also, stay away from the foods listed in the "Types of foods to avoid" section earlier, and manage your stress. Stress can cause inflammation that disrupts your gut microbiome. Those little bugs are super-responsive to what you put in your body and how you feel! They even help keep depression at bay.

What's on the menu: specific foods for hormone balance

This is your quick reference list of what to eat! Make trips to the grocery store easy on yourself—go ahead and copy this directly onto your shopping list. I've also included some easy ways to actually eat these foods. You don't have to be a Michelin star chef to eat delicious, healthy meals.

- **Nuts and seeds:** Eat nuts and seeds as a snack on their own, add them to salads, or make a rich, spreadable butter. You can also roast them in the oven with your favorite spices for a crunchy snack. Try cinnamon, sesame, or jalapeno!
- **Avocados:** Avocados can be sliced and added to sandwiches or salads, mashed, and used as a spread. They give smoothies a nice creamy texture. They also make a great substitute for butter or oil in baking recipes.
- **Flaxseeds:** Grind them up and add them to smoothies for a boost of fiber and healthy fats. Vegans love them as a good egg substitute (in baking recipes, not omelets!).
- **Quinoa:** Cook it like rice and use it as a base for salads or grain bowls. I love using quinoa as a substitute for rice or pasta.

- **Chickpeas:** Chickpeas are yummy when you roast them with your favorite seasonings. Eat them for a crunchy snack or add them to salads for a boost of protein. Try making homemade hummus or blending them into soups for a creamy texture.
- **Salmon and fatty fish:** Salmon and other fatty fish can be baked, grilled, or broiled with your favorite seasonings for a healthy and delicious meal. You can also add them to salads or use them to make fish tacos.
- **Chicken and poultry:** Chicken and other poultry are delicious baked, grilled, or sautéed with your favorite seasonings. They can also be added to salads or used in stir-fry recipes.
- **Grass-fed organic red meat:** Grill it, bake it, broil it, sauté it, love it! Serve choice cuts with sauces, or make burgers, pasta dishes, casseroles, salads, stir-fries, tacos, sandwiches, and more.
- **Eggs:** A classic breakfast food for a good reason! Eggs can be scrambled, fried, or boiled. They're quick to cook and delicious. You can also hard-boil them and add them to salads, or just reach for one when you need a quick protein-rich snack.
- **Whole fruits:** Whole fruits are great snacks! I especially like cherries and pomegranates for hormone balance. Eat them whole, slice them up, and serve them on a salad, add them to smoothies, make jam, or dry them to snack on during a hike.

(You can also use them to make fruit juice but try not to do this too often. Fruit juice gives you all of a fruit's sugars but none of the important fiber.)

- **Kale, cauliflower, and broccoli:** Roast them or sauté them with your favorite seasonings. Of course, they're perfect for salads, but they're also great when you add them to soups and stews . . . or even as pizza toppings!
- **Kombucha, kimchi, and sauerkraut:** Gut-friendly probiotics! They're delicious by themselves, but they work well in smoothies, too. Kimchi and sauerkraut spice up dishes they're added to. Just keep in mind that cooking them will kill off the good bacteria you want for your gut health, so try to use them in raw recipes or add them after the rest of the ingredients have cooked and cooled down.
- **Coconut milk or goat milk:** Just because you're avoiding the hormones in dairy, doesn't mean you don't get a creamy drink. Coconut milk and goat milk are delicious. Use them just like dairy milk, alone or in recipes.
- **Spices, especially turmeric and cinnamon:** I could never list all the ways to use spices in a quick paragraph! They're too delicious and versatile. That said, these particular spices taste great added to smoothies for a boost of flavor and health benefits. They're also yummy on roasted

vegetables or blended into homemade spice blends.

Supplements for hormone balance

If you decide to take supplements, make sure you buy from a reliable company. I hate to say it, but a lot of supplement companies sell bad products. Supplements are either adulterated (when cheaper, less effective stuff is added to the real thing), or they're flat-out not what they claim to be. Either way, they're probably not "organic" or "natural" like the labels say. Those words have unfortunately become marketing terms, in most cases.

A few companies I like are Standard Process, Pure Encapsulations, and Thorne.

Which supplements should you consider taking?

- **Progesterone cream:** The #1 hormone-repair product! If you make no other changes, I hope you'll start using progesterone cream. For some people, making this one change transforms their health so dramatically, they don't need to do much else.
- **Magnesium:** Magnesium is the hormone-healing mineral! Almost every woman who struggles with her period or menopause could use a good magnesium supplement. It plays a crucial role in over 300 processes in the body. It gives you the building blocks for healthy hormones, including

progesterone.[71] It's right up there with progesterone cream for products I recommend to almost everyone.

- **Zinc:** Zinc may raise the number of binding sites on your progesterone receptors.[72]
- **Vitamin D:** You've heard of the "sunshine vitamin," right? Vitamin D is critical for hormone balance. It helps regulate estrogen, progesterone, and testosterone. Vitamin D deficiency has been linked to hormone-related health issues like polycystic ovary syndrome (PCOS) and infertility.[73]
- **Omega-3 fatty acids:** Another key building block for hormone production! These are the healthy fats that reduce inflammation and improve insulin sensitivity.
- **Vitamin C:** This antioxidant reduces oxidative stress and inflammation, both of which can contribute to hormonal imbalances. Vitamin C is also important for the production of adrenal hormones, such as cortisol. In studies, women who took vitamin C had higher progesterone levels and higher pregnancy rates.[74]
- **Liver-support nutrients:** The liver plays a critical role in hormone metabolism and elimination. So supporting your liver with nutrients such as milk thistle, Livaplex by Standard Process, and dandelion root can help heal your hormones.

- **Probiotics:** If you don't want to add more pre- and probiotics into your diet, you can find a good pill-based supplement. A lot of probiotic supplements need to be refrigerated to preserve the living bacteria. But you can find high-quality shelf-stable options that will be perfectly fine in your pantry or medicine cabinet. Supplementing with probiotics can help restore the balance of gut bacteria, which is one of the key players in creating a healthy endocrine system and overall wellness.
- **B Vitamins:** B vitamins, including B6, B12, and folate, are important for hormone metabolism and production.[75] They also help reduce stress and improve energy levels.
- **Fiber:** You want your gut to be nice and balanced, so your poops are regularly eliminating estrogen from your system.

Herbs to balance your progesterone

If you're going to use herbs for hormone balance, I don't recommend using too many at the same time. Herbs are powerful; they can have drug-like effects on the body and they don't all play well together. Talk to a certified herbalist or an expert who can help you choose the right one (or a few).

- **Chasteberry (*Vitex agnus-castus*)** – This one is so popular that it's often lovingly referred to as

simply "Vitex." Vitex helps regulate your period and balance your hormones. It works by lowering your prolactin levels.[76] Since prolactin can interrupt your progesterone production, balancing it has a powerful effect.
- **Red raspberry leaf (*Rubus idaeus*)** – Red raspberry is another classic! The leaves contain phyto-progesterone. It helps regulate your period, protect your uterus for childbearing and birth, reduce fibroids, reduce fluid retention, and tone your pelvic floor.
- **Bupleurum (*Bupleurum falcatum*)** – This herb mimics progesterone in your body, making it a great choice for balancing your estrogen levels.[77]
- **White peony (*Paeonia lactiflora*)** – White peony has been shown to boost your natural progesterone production (but be aware as it can also reduce testosterone levels).[77] It's excellent if you have irregular periods or really bad cramps. (But if you have period flooding or menorrhagia, you might want to choose another herb.)

Other herbs that deserve a mention are Kenya oak (*Vitex fischeri*, from the same plant genus as chasteberry), dill (*Anethum graveolens*, and yup—it's the same dill you have in your kitchen!), and maca root (*Lepidium meyenii*, a cruciferous veggie and adaptogen that helps balance your hormone levels over time).

STRESS

Stress is the killer of all!

We've already talked multiple times about how your stress response is activated and why it's important for your safety. You've also learned that stress hormones, like cortisol, are important if you don't want to nod off at work or sleep through your kid's dance recital. (I know, it's boring when your kid's not on the stage. But you don't want her to catch you snoozing!)

So cortisol and a little stress are important.

But you know what happens if stress becomes chronic. Now you're dealing with anxiety (and maybe even depression). It throws everything off: your sleep, energy levels, mental clarity, immune system, sex drive, mood, and yes, your hormones. Even if everything else in your body is working like a beautiful handmade Swiss clock, stress can be enough to throw a wrench in the entire system.

Remember the story about my hives?

A long period of stress triggered that condition. And later, it was a stressful event (a phone call) that started my period when I thought I was postmenopausal. Sure, that period flushed out all the hormones that were causing my hives and led me to the understanding that my autoimmunity was hormone-based. That understanding was a happy side effect. It still shouldn't be ignored that stress was powerful enough to trigger a period in a postmenopausal woman.

The good news is, there are a lot of ways you can combat stress and support your hormones.

I'll touch on a few here: mindfulness meditation and orgasm. (Yup—orgasm!)

What about pharmaceuticals for anxiety and depression? I'm not going to tell someone who is seriously struggling with their mental health not to take drugs. It's not easy to treat depression and anxiety 100% naturally. Sometimes life puts a difficult decision in front of you. Make the choice you feel is best for yourself. If you choose to take the pills, please understand that they're disrupting your body's ability to make its own natural hormones. Do what you can to support your natural hormones in other ways.

Mindfulness meditation

You don't have to live at an ashram to practice meditation. You don't even have to be good at clearing your mind. If the word "meditation" inspires a knee-jerk reaction of "I can't do that," then just think of it as paying attention. That's all mindfulness meditation is, really. Learn to harness the power of your attention, and you'll learn to give more attention to the things that make you feel good. Mindfulness is about focusing your attention on the present moment, without judgment or distraction.

Are you thinking, *"C'mon, Liz. Meditation? My problems are serious. How much of a difference can meditation make?"*

That depends. I know people who say it doesn't work at all and others who healed their depression and transformed their entire lives with mindfulness. One thing is for sure:

mountains of research show the benefits of regularly practicing mindfulness.

The American Psychological Association says:

> "Psychologists have found that mindfulness meditation changes our brain and biology in positive ways, improving mental and physical health . . .

> "Researchers reviewed more than 200 studies of mindfulness among healthy people and found mindfulness-based therapy was especially effective for reducing stress, anxiety and depression. Mindfulness can also help treat people with specific problems including depression, pain, smoking and addiction. Some of the most promising research has looked at people with depression. Several studies have found, for example, that MBCT [mindfulness-based cognitive therapy] can significantly reduce relapse in people who have had previous episodes of major depression. What's more, mindfulness-based interventions can improve physical health, too. For example, mindfulness may reduce pain, fatigue and stress in people with chronic pain. Other studies have found preliminary evidence that mindfulness might boost the immune system and help people recover more quickly from cold or flu."[78]

Pretty big claims! But they're not unfounded. Mindfulness can lower cortisol, raise serotonin, ease insomnia, and even cool down hot flashes.[78]

If you have trouble focusing your attention, try joining a yoga or meditation class. I'm not saying yoga will help heal your stress or depression. But it can help you learn to focus your attention. (And yoga itself is great for your hormones, so you're killing two birds with one stone!)

Orgasm

A lot of people perk up when I talk about this one!

If your hormones are out of whack, then you might find it harder to orgasm—if you have a libido at all. But orgasms are important for your hormone balance and overall well-being. Why? Because orgasms release oxytocin.

Oxytocin is the "feel good" hormone. It makes you feel warm, fuzzy, and just plain happy all over. But oxytocin's job doesn't stop there. Oxytocin is required for contractions during childbirth. It's essential for lactation. It reduces stress, insomnia, breast cancer, and stress-related illnesses (including gut problems like IBS) and supports your cognitive functions. It suppresses inflammation and supports your immune health. It inhibits your appetite and reduces obesity. It even has mild antibiotic effects to help prevent infections (especially uterine infections). It sparks your curiosity and keeps you hungry to learn new things, even priming pathways in your brain to help you absorb new knowledge.[79,80]

Oxytocin also helps balance your other hormones. It tells your hypothalamus to create a hormone called LHRH.

LHRH then goes to your pituitary gland and tells it to release LH (luteinizing hormone) and FSH (follicle-stimulating hormone).[81] That's how oxytocin plays a role in your fertility.

One way I like to explain oxytocin is that it resets all your other hormones.

Even when your hormones are healthy, they fluctuate a lot—especially during your childbearing years. Your body knows that fluctuating, unbalanced hormones can be a recipe for a health disaster. So oxytocin helps keep your entire endocrine system aligned. How does your body ensure you get a steady supply of oxytocin?

It has a natural "reset" button: your clitoris!

A clitoral orgasm releases a flood of oxytocin through your body, triggering all the balancing benefits I just mentioned. Now there's something your doctor won't tell you! Most doctors will say the clitoris serves no purpose on the body. They think it's completely unnecessary apart from pleasure (as if pleasure was unnecessary!). That couldn't be further from the truth!

Craving the pleasure keeps you reaching for your clitoris, resetting your hormones each time you reach orgasm. Have you ever been sick and found that you had insatiable cravings for fruit? That's your body naturally reaching out for the glucose and vitamins in the fruit. It knows what it needs. Your craving for pleasure and orgasm is the same.

(By the way, this is totally different from how a man understands orgasm. As men think of it, orgasm is related to ejaculation and conception. Ejaculation and orgasm are actually two different events in a man's body, but they usually happen at the same time. So in his mind "orgasm = ejaculation = baby-making." They're all the same event. That's why, for such a long time, men thought that the female orgasm was necessary for conception, too.)

Have you ever met up with one of your friends and thought, *Wow, she looks amazing! It's like she's glowing! What is she doing?* When you mention how good she looks, she says, "Oh, I have a new boyfriend . . . and we're having lots of great sex!" You congratulate her, but secretly think, *Yeah, right! I bet she just went on a diet.*

Well, sorry to burst your bubble, but she's telling the truth. It's the sex! All that oxytocin is flowing through her, giving her all the health benefits I mentioned earlier. It's got her feeling so healthy and happy that she seems to glow from within.

Great orgasms are more than a luxury. They're essential!

If you're on the birth control pill or HRT, I'm not surprised if your sex drive is lagging . . . or dead altogether. Synthetic hormones downregulate your oxytocin receptors. Because your receptors are less sensitive, your body thinks it needs more of the hormone. Soon, you've got an oxytocin overload, yet you're not getting any of the benefits! It's like an addiction; the more you take a drug, the more of it you need to get the same effects.

This is bad news for your sex life and your relationship overall.

You might say, "*But Liz, if women on the pill and HRT have higher levels of oxytocin, surely that means they have even more of its benefits!*"

Sorry, but it doesn't work that way.

A 2015 study looked at whether oxytocin could make women feel more in love when they looked at their partner's face. That's one thing oxytocin is supposed to do. It's supposed to give you a rush of love for your romantic partner and make you think they're more beautiful than any other person. In this study, researchers gave oxytocin to two groups of women: one group who was not on the birth control pill, and another group who was. The group *not* on the pill experienced the expected response. When they were on the oxytocin and shown a picture of their partner's face, they went, *Ooh la la! What a honey!*

The group who did take the pill experienced . . . crickets.

> "*[In women who were **not** using hormonal contraceptives, aka HC] . . . treatment with oxytocin increased the perceived attractiveness of the partner relative to other men, which was paralleled by elevated responses in reward-associated regions . . . These effects of oxytocin were absent in women using HC.*"[82]

Ouch! It breaks my heart to see women on synthetic hormones not understanding why they don't feel in love with their partners anymore. They don't have a libido, they can't reach orgasm as easily, and their bodies can't access the hormone that makes them feel in love.

So what can you do to increase your oxytocin?

Masturbate or have sex! Start the day out right: with an orgasm. It'll set you up for hormonal and emotional success for the rest of the day. You might want to get a good vibrator. Suction vibrators work wonders. Don't shy away from using them with your partner, too. Toys should add to your bedroom experience, not replace your partner.

Eat fruits, avocado, sashimi, and raw Brazil nuts. (Whatever they say about oysters, the little mollusks certainly don't increase *female* libido! Men may like their appearance, though.)

Try to manage your stress. Oxytocin can help relieve stress, but too much stress wrecks your libido (even for masturbation). That traps you in a cycle of high-stress-no-sex. Not a fun cycle to ride!

Set aside regular time for it in your schedule. Take your time, especially if you've been having trouble reaching orgasm or if you've never had one. (If that sounds familiar, you're not alone! A lot of women reach their first orgasm around age 18, but some don't orgasm until their 40s!) It's no good demanding "It's time to orgasm . . . now! I don't have all day!" Be patient with yourself. Make sure you create a comfy, romantic atmosphere, and learn what your body likes. Indulge in a lot of fun fantasies, too.

Some men feel confused when it comes to helping a woman orgasm. Here are a few tips:

- **Don't just dive into sex:** Warm her up with love, romance, cuddling, and compliments. Tell her she's beautiful and sexy! She wants to know that you want her.
- **Ask her what she wants:** Don't be nervous or proud about it. Encourage her to tell you what she wants more of and what's not working.
- **Caress her breasts:** Some women learn to come from breast stimulation alone.
- **Show her clitoris some love:** Remember that her clitoris is the center of her pleasure. This is where her orgasm comes from. This is the part of her body that would have turned into her penis if she had been a male. She probably won't have an orgasm if you don't stimulate her clitoris.
- **Give her oral sex:** Most women adore oral sex, and some even say they can't come if they don't receive it.

EXERCISE

Your relationship with your body is the closest, most personal relationship you'll ever have. Your body will be with you until the very end! I'm a big proponent of loving your body just as it is.

Personally, I hate exercising . . . and shame on me! That said, I understand how important it is. So every morning, after I wake up and before I have breakfast, I exercise for 10 minutes. And I go hard! I get my heart rate up until I'm huffing and puffing.

I also practice intermittent fasting. My preferred style is to stop eating at about three o'clock every day. That means when I wake up in the morning, I'm coming off of an 18- to 20-hour fast. My hard-charging morning exercise now forces me to burn calories from body fat, not from food. This boosts my metabolism for the entire day. But that's far from the only benefit my quick, 10-minute daily routine gets me.

Exercise is just plain good for you in every way: physically, mentally, and emotionally. It helps you reach and maintain a healthy weight, strengthens and builds your muscles, creates stronger bones, reduces your risk of chronic disease, supports immunity, and even helps keep your endocrine system balanced.

One study, published in the journal *Breast Cancer Research*, found that women who regularly exercised had higher levels of SHBG, which is a substance that binds to estrogen and testosterone, stopping them from circulating through the body.[83] That's just one way exercise balances your hormones. Another way is by reducing your body fat. Body fat stores estrogen (and creates it). Decrease your body fat, and you can lower your estrogen levels.

Plus, exercise is great for your self-esteem. The more you do it, the healthier you get, and the better you look! It's a big boost when you glimpse yourself in the mirror before stepping into the shower and think, *"Wow . . . is that muscle definition in my arms? I'm lookin' good!"*

How often should you exercise? The rule of thumb is: if you're doing nothing, do something. If you're doing something, do more. The only exception to this is if you're a serious athlete and training all the time, in which case your body fat and cholesterol may be too low to make healthy hormones.

Any kind of movement is better than nothing. Even gardening or cleaning your house is better than binge-watching TV on the sofa!

Low-intensity exercises, like yoga and Pilates, strengthen and tone your body, while helping you develop mental clarity. Yoga in particular is great for lowering stress. There's also a type of training called "Zone 2." It involves working out at low intensity for a longer period of time (like walking for an hour). Zone 2 supports your mitochondria, and reduces your risk of heart disease, cancer, metabolic syndrome, and more.

Weight training builds muscles and reduces fat. You should immediately try lifting the biggest weights at the gym every day until you can do it, and then enter one of those muscle competitions where people wear bathing suits and oil up their muscles.

Just kidding! Start small, with weights that start to feel too heavy after 10 reps or so. At first, you'll think, *"These aren't too heavy. I've got this!"* But after those 10 reps, you'll feel the burn. That's lactic acid building in your muscles. It means your muscles are growing.

Don't be afraid of high-intensity exercise, either. HIIT training (high-intensity interval training) conditions your heart, strengthens muscles and bones, builds stamina, and burns tons of fat!

There are so many different ways to exercise, I know you can find something that makes you want to move. If you'd like to get out and make friends, try joining a fitness class, dance class, or hiking group. If you don't like people, get a gym membership, or follow online workouts.

Carve out some space in your life for fitness. Studies show that people who exercise in the mornings tend to stick with their workout routines because it happens at a regular time during the day. Like an orgasm, starting your day with a workout sets you up for long-term health. If you do it in the morning, you get it out of the way and then you can go about your life.

SLEEP

Your sleep and your hormones are so closely connected, it's not easy to know which came first: sleep problems or hormone problems.

Either way, getting better sleep will definitely have a positive effect on your hormones.

During sleep, your body releases HGH. It helps rebuild damaged tissues, heal your cells, and repair your muscles. So if you're not sleeping, your cells aren't repairing themselves very well. That's part of why a lot of sleepless nights make you look older. Your skin literally hasn't had a chance to repair itself from daily damage! But this isn't about vanity. The problem of slow (or low) cell repair is more than skin-deep. If your skin cells aren't repairing or regenerating, neither are cells through the rest of your body.

Sleep also downregulates cortisone, calming stress. It activates your immune system, reducing inflammation, pain, and infection. It makes sure your body produces melatonin (the "I'm feeling sleepy" hormone) on a regular, reliable schedule. Otherwise, your body will be confused about how much melatonin to make and when to make it.

Progesterone has a sleep-inducing effect at bedtime. If it's not present, guess what? Neither is sleep. Here are some tips for sleeping like a baby:

- **Stick to a regular sleep schedule:** Try to go to bed and wake up at the same time every day, even on weekends.
- **Create a relaxing sleep environment:** Make sure your bedroom is dark, cool, and quiet. Use comfortable pillows and a supportive mattress. Don't use your bed for anything other than sleep and sex.
- **Avoid exercise right before bedtime:** Exercise endorphins get energy flowing through your brain and make you want to stay up.

- **Avoid screens before bedtime:** Try to avoid using electronic devices such as smartphones, tablets, or laptops before bed.
- **View sunlight immediately after waking up:** This tells your body, "Look, that's the sun! It's time to wake up!" and your body starts producing cortisol. (Just enough to wake you up and spark your energy.)
- **Create a relaxing bedtime routine:** Take a warm bath, read a book, do yoga, or listen to calming music before bed.
- **No caffeine or alcohol:** It probably doesn't surprise you that caffeine keeps you awake. But alcohol, which most people think of as a nervous system depressant, can keep you up, too. That's because alcohol is both a depressant and a stimulant. It might make you tired at first, but later in the night, it disrupts your REM cycle. So your sleep will be restless, or you'll wake up at 3 a.m. No thanks!
- **Get regular exercise:** Exercise during the day can help improve sleep quality.
- **Have an orgasm:** The reason you feel super sleepy after orgasms is because of all that juicy oxytocin flooding your system. Having an orgasm at bedtime might be just what the doctor ordered. (Not that most doctors will actually recommend this . . . although they should!)

ENVIRONMENTAL TOXINS

So far, we've talked about ways you can balance your hormones from within. Diet, supplements, exercise, stress, and sleep—these all work with your endocrine system by creating change within the internal environment of your body.

Now it's time to talk about reducing your exposure to external toxins. *Let's stop endocrine disruptors from getting into your body in the first place.*

When I help people create hormone healing plans, this is one of the areas where I get the most pushback.

Okay, there's usually pushback in multiple areas! Most people find the idea of changing their habits pretty unappealing. They have to eat healthier, heal their gut, exercise, have more orgasms, reduce their stress, *and* purge their homes of xenoestrogen? That's way too much! Can't they just balance their hormones by popping a pill or something?

Doctors will tell you it works like that. Most of them actually believe it's true. They believe you can skip all of this by just taking synthetic hormones—the pill or HRT. But now you know that synthetic hormones come with a whole host of health problems, and they don't protect you from xenoestrogens.

You can absolutely do this! Millions of women just like you have done it. I've done it myself. Take things one step at a time. Think of it as an adventure. This book is your permission slip to try a bunch of new things: new foods, new exercises, new products, and new homemade recipes! It feels like you're changing your life . . . *because you are changing your life!*

It's important to take action if you can. Even if you do everything I suggest in this book, our world is still full of xenoestrogens. They're in your furniture, carpets, and in the stores and restaurants you go to. They're in the water and air. They're pretty hard to avoid. Changing the products you use is important if you want to reduce your exposure.

Ready to learn how to get endocrine disruptors out of your home?

Replace your cleaning products

Most cleaning products sold in stores are swimming with endocrine disruptors.

Visit the cleaning aisle of your grocery store, and the harsh chemical smell greets you like a kick to the face. Sometimes just walking down that aisle can make my eyes water. Pick up a bottle and check the label, and you'll find a long list of hard-to-pronounce chemical ingredients, as well as a loud danger warning that makes your eyes bug out of your head. Why would you want to clean your home with something that can cause respiratory issues and includes known endocrine disruptors? Yup! The companies use ingredients that are well known to cause endocrine issues! What do they care about if they can save a buck?

The good news is that our grandmothers had no problem cleaning their homes without all those specialized, chemical-laden products. They used a few simple ingredients that work to cut grime and kill germs.

It's a myth that modern society is cleaner and healthier because the chemical products we've created are better at cutting dirt and killing germs. Modern society is cleaner and healthier because we understand the importance of cleanliness.

It's even a myth that you need antibacterial soaps and cleaners.[84] Today's scientists are actually worried about how popular antibacterial cleaners are. Why? Look at the label of an antibacterial cleaner. Does it say, "Kills 99.9% of bacteria?" Sounds pretty good, doesn't it? Yeah, that's what generations of scientists thought, too. But the .1% of bacteria that didn't die turned out to be super-bacteria that were immune to the chemicals in the cleaner. That super-bacteria proliferated. Now we've got a world full of super-bacteria that we can't kill with popular antibacterials.[84] (Some scientists have a real problem with long-term thinking, huh?)

The natural ingredients I'm about to share work just as well at killing bacteria (or washing them away so they don't cause problems), and they don't lead to "superbugs." Here are some of the products your grandmother used, which you can use too:

- **High-proof alcohol:** Kills germs and bacteria! Surprisingly, 70% isopropyl alcohol is more effective at killing germs than 90%. You can also use Everclear.

- **White vinegar:** White vinegar is acidic. It cuts through grime, dirt, grease, and mineral deposits. It also kills bacteria.
- **Castile soap:** It's soap. It washes away dirt, grime, and pretty much anything else you want to clean.
- **Baking soda:** Looking for a gritty scrubbing effect? Use baking soda to scrub your sinks, tub, and tiles.

If the list looks short, that's because it is. You don't need a closet full of specialized products. You can mix and match most of these ingredients to make your own safe, natural products for every room in your house. Get yourself some basic supplies, like spray bottles, sponges or brushes, microfiber cloths, and maybe some pure, organic essential oils to scent your cleaning products. A lot of essential oils have natural germ-fighting activities, like tea tree (*Melaleuca alternifolia*) and lemongrass (*Cymbopogon citratus*). Stay away from fragrance oils, though—those are synthetic.

Here are a few simple recipes to get you started:

All-Purpose Cleaner

Mix 1 part white vinegar with 1 part water in a spray bottle. If you want to make a sanitizing cleaner, add ½ part high-proof alcohol. (So if you've got 1 cup white vinegar and 1 cup water, you'd add ½ cup high-proof alcohol.)

Tub & Tile Scrub

Mix baking soda, castile soap, and water to make a paste. Adjust the texture by adding more baking soda (to make it thicker), or one of the liquid ingredients to make it more liquidy. The baking soda creates the scrubby action, and the castile soap lifts dirt.

Apply the paste to the tub, let it sit for 15 minutes, then scrub with a sponge or brush. Rinse.

Glass Cleaner

Mix 1 part white vinegar with 1 part water in a spray bottle.

Spray the solution onto glass surfaces and wipe with a cloth or paper towel.

Toilet Cleaner

Mix 1 cup of baking soda with 1 cup of white vinegar.

Pour the mixture into the toilet bowl and let it sit for 10 to 15 minutes. Scrub the bowl with a toilet brush and flush.

Carpet & Upholstery Freshener

Mix 1/2 cup baking soda with a few drops of your favorite essential oil.

Sprinkle the mixture onto carpets or upholstery. Let it sit for 15 to 20 minutes and then vacuum it up.

Replace your personal care products

Your skin does an excellent job of keeping toxins out of your body. But it's not an impenetrable barrier. It's permeable. Think of your skin as a thick membrane that absorbs some things and allows them into your body. That's how some topical medications and natural progesterone cream work.

But it's also why an alarming number of body products and cosmetics introduce xenoestrogens into your body—

where they disrupt your endocrine system, cause cancer, and even lead to genetic mutations.

Almost every commercial body product you find at the drugstore falls into the danger zone. They're treated with chemicals to make them smell good (synthetic fragrances), give them a smooth or lathery texture, and preserve their shelf lives. The FDA has decided these chemicals are okay. Either they haven't gotten around to doing research on the individual chemicals (of which there are hundreds, if not thousands!), or they've decided the research doesn't show enough of a risk.

I'm going to ask you to guess how many of these chemicals the FDA has actually banned. For reference, the EU has banned over 1,600 chemicals from cosmetics. So how many do you think the US has banned?

As I'm writing this book, the answer is nine.[85]

Yup. Just nine.

California, Maryland, and Colorado are a little ahead of the curve. California and Maryland prohibit 24 chemicals from use in cosmetics, while California and Colorado have banned "forever chemicals," like PFAs.[85] ("Forever chemicals" don't biodegrade. Once they're created, they're around forever. When you use them, they get into your body . . . and if your body manages to successfully detox them, the chemicals enter the environment. And there they stay forever, polluting waterways and soil, disrupting the biology of wildlife and plants, and just generally making an eternal nuisance of themselves.)

How can cosmetic companies get away with this? Because consumers want cheap products that last a long time, and corporate lobbyists have a lot of influence over the government.

Thankfully, a lot of consumers recognize the problem and are demanding cleaner products. Every year, more products come on the market that aren't saturated with endocrine disruptors. Find a few organic, green brands you trust, like Tata Harper, Honest Beauty, and Love Beauty & Planet.

It's also easier than you might think to make your own products at home.

Try using pure, organic argan oil (*Argania spinosa*) and shea butter (*Vitellaria paradoxa*) to moisturize, make beeswax (*Cera flava*) balms to stop the skin from losing moisture, and use aloe vera (*Aloe barbadensis*) to heal irritated skin. Those are just a few examples, of course. There are dozens (if not hundreds) of natural oils, butters, and kitchen ingredients you can use for skin and body care.

Gardening products

Maybe what you put into your garden doesn't seem like that big of a deal. After all, these products aren't going directly on your skin. They're not even going into your house (unless you have house plants). They're going into the soil outside.

But that means the ground around your home is literally full of endocrine disruptors. Some of them will evaporate into the air around your living space. If you grow herbs, fruits, or vegetables, guess what? Those xenoestrogens are in your beautiful homegrown food.

As much as possible, use organic gardening products, like potting soil, fertilizers, and pesticides.

Plastic

This is a tough one for a lot of people! It's one thing to buy natural cleaning products and make a face scrub out of brown sugar and avocado oil. It's another thing to stop buying food that's packaged in plastic, avoid getting take-out that comes in plastic or Styrofoam containers, get rid of plastic Tupperware and leftover containers, stop buying plastic bottles (including bottled water), skip the plastic toys for your kids, and just try to stop using plastic in your life as much as possible.

I get it! It seems like *everything* contains plastic these days! How did it become so ubiquitous?

Plastic was first created in the 1800s. But just like synthetic hormones and endocrine-disrupting chemicals, plastic really took off after WWII. Using plastics instead of wood made furniture more affordable. Using them to make car parts made owning a car possible for the average family. Replacing glass with plastic in the kitchen made it less likely that a bottle would break if you dropped it . . . and meant you didn't have to stop cooking dinner to clean up broken glass!

As usual, scientists applauded themselves for saving the world, without realizing the damage they were causing.

As of 2023, plastic production has ballooned from 5

million metric tons in 1950 to 380 million metric tons.[86] This is having a disastrous impact on our environment and our health. Think about this: all of the plastic that has ever been produced still exists in one form or another. It can't be completely broken down and biodegraded. It can take hundreds of years for a piece of plastic to break down . . . and even then, it's just dissolved into teeny-tiny particles of plastic! These teeny-tiny "microplastics" fill our oceans and the fish within them. They contaminate our soil, air, plants, wildlife, our own bodies, and those of our children. Did you know that microplastics have even been detected in the bodies of fetuses in the womb? It's absolutely heartbreaking.

For those who believe this pollution isn't having an effect on our health, I can only point to the rampant rates of cancer and endocrine disorders afflicting our society.

Are you saying, *"But Liz, I recycle my plastic!"*

Well, that sounds responsible. There was a time when scientists believed recycling plastic would be the answer. But now it's clear that, while recycling paper, glass, and metal is working pretty well, recycling plastics just doesn't work.[87] There are too many different chemical formulas for plastic. These plastics may all look like the same thing to the average consumer, but they're very different products. They can't all be broken down and recycled. They can't be recombined with one another.

I know it's going to be tough, if not impossible, to reduce your use of plastics. But I encourage you to do your best. It may seem like an inconvenient choice with small rewards, but I promise it has huge benefits for your health, your family's health, and the health of our planet. And because it's unlikely the government is going to take any meaningful action to stop the plastic plague, the best action happens with you and me.

Consider where you live

Do you live in a heavily polluted city? Or downriver from a factory that pumps toxic waste into the water? Or near a factory where combustion fills the air with clouds of benzene and dioxins? Or maybe you live near farmlands that are treated with chemicals, and these seep into your drinking water?

You might want to think about moving.

Decades of horror movies have warned you against building your home on an ancient Native American burial ground. (Nobody needs the stress of annoyed ghosts slamming open their kitchen cabinets all night!) Just so, you might not want to live on land that's polluted with endocrine-disrupting chemicals. I'll take the ghosts any day!

DAILY SCHEDULE FOR HORMONE BALANCE

In the morning

- Wake up naturally with the sun if you can or use an alarm clock that slowly gets louder (instead of jarring yourself out of a deep sleep with a sudden loud buzzing noise).

- Take in some sunlight for about 15 minutes. Your body says to itself, "It's the sun! It must be time to wake up!" This jumpstarts your body's daily cortisol production and gets your energy flowing. If you can't view sunlight, turn up the lights in your room.
- While taking in the light, drink a whole glass of water. Drinking water before putting anything else in your stomach helps detox your body, rehydrates you after sleep, supports your bowel movements, and more.
- Time for an orgasm! Hop back into bed and masturbate or have sex until you orgasm. Give yourself a healthy flow of oxytocin to reset your hormones that may have become imbalanced and reduce your stress levels.
- Eat a light breakfast. Go for something rich in fiber or choose a protein like Greek yogurt with nuts, eggs, or lox on flaxseed crackers.
- Meditate and do your fitness practice. Starting with meditation gives your body time to digest your food, so you'll be less likely to get nauseous when you're working out.

Afternoon

- Eat lunch. Go for hormone-friendly carbs (flaxseed crackers or quinoa), rich fats (avocado),

lean protein (chicken or fish), and plenty of green veggies. Don't forget your probiotics (kombucha or sauerkraut)!
- Take a walk after lunch to support your digestion and work off excess energy from any carbs you ate.
- If your energy starts to slump a few hours after lunch, eat a light snack of protein and fiber. Try homemade granola bars, veggies and hummus, or nut butter on rice crackers.

Evening

- Eat your dinner about 3 hours after your snack . . . and remember to fill your plate with mostly veggies and protein.
- When the sun sets, turn off blue light and turn down the lights in your home to signal to your body that it's time to get ready for sleep. Cortisol production tapers off, and your body starts producing melatonin. If you have a dimmer switch, that's great!
- Start your bedtime routine, whether it includes reading, meditation, or a warm bath or shower.
- Go to bed around 3 hours after dinner. This gives your body time to digest your food, without leaving you time to get hungry again before bed.
- Sweet dreams!

YOUR PATH TO HEALING

For millennia, women turned to their mothers, aunts, and grandmothers for wisdom and remedies. We passed on the knowledge of which plants promoted fertility, healthy pregnancy, and regular periods. We ushered each other through menopause with herbs that kept our health stable even as our hormones fluctuated. Women's knowledge was a sacred practice handed down from generation to generation.

The cycle was interrupted when men took over all aspects of medicine, shutting women out, and drug companies concocted chemicals to "cure" us and make themselves rich. Whether they knew what they were doing or not, they sold us lies. We've paid the price with our health and happiness.

Your symptoms, whatever they are, are not your fault. Our entire world is chemically altered with endocrine disruptors, and it only seems to be getting worse (xenoestrogens have a whole generation of young people confused about their gender). When we get sick as a result, drug companies would have us believe that more chemicals are the answer. It sounds audacious to say that even Western medicine's most talented, educated, passionate doctors don't understand the problem—but it's true. If you've been struggling with mysterious health problems or hormone issues, you've experienced that truth for yourself.

But the knowledge of the past is still with us, though it's been buried. Women can turn to each other for the wisdom to reclaim their health. You might have to dig a little and talk to some healers on the so-called "fringe" of society, like homeopaths, functional nutritionists, and people who run vitamin shops, but the fact that you read this book means you're already on your own path of healing. Use the knowledge in this book. Start using natural progesterone cream today and implement any other suggestions that you can. As you heal yourself, you put yourself in a position to help other women who don't know where to turn—and the men and children in your life, too.

If you have questions, contact me through my website.

Healing others is one of my greatest passions! I'll be honored to serve you as a consultant and teacher. Together, we'll get to the root of your symptoms and create a plan of action to bring you back to peak health and happiness.

Contact me through my website and join my email list to stay updated on natural health information, new books, and other specials. My URL is HealthyLivingByLiz.com, or you can scan the QR code below.

Thank you for caring about your health and being part of the solution!

ABOUT THE AUTHOR

Liz Herzog is a certified naturopath with over 20 years of experience working in and owning natural health shops. Over this time period, she worked one-on-one with hundreds of customers who didn't find answers in Western medicine. She is certified to teach about nutrition and alternative medicine (but not to treat patients).

As she helped her customers heal with natural remedies, Liz came to realize that many health issues—especially women's issues—are rooted in hormonal imbalance. Her understanding deepened after struggling with her own illness, including a serious case of hives that lasted five years and left her doctors stumped. That ordeal and healing process taught her that hormonal imbalance can have system-wide consequences on the whole body, creating a domino effect of symptoms that seem unrelated. But, as Liz likes to say, "We are walking hormones! Your hormones run you."

Liz is also a specialist in gut health, and other natural health topics, and continues to help clients on a private basis through her website at HealthyLivingByLiz.com. She lives in California close to her two sons and their families.

REFERENCES

1. Endocrine System. Cleveland Clinic. May 12, 2020. Accessed on May 11, 2023. https://my.clevelandclinic.org/health/articles/21201-endocrine-system
2. What Are the Different Types of Estrogen? Tyson's Gynecology. Accessed on May 11, 2023. https://www.tysonsgynecology.com/what-are-the-different-types-of-estrogen/
3. Endocrine Disorders: Causes & Treatment. Tampa General Hospital. Accessed on May 11, 2023. https://www.tgh.org/institutes-and-services/conditions/endocrine-disorder
4. Estrogen's Effects on the Female Body. Johns Hopkins Medicine. Accessed on May 11, 2023. https://www.hopkinsmedicine.org/health/conditions-and-diseases/estrogens-effects-on-the-female-body
5. Breast Cancer Risk: Menopausal Hormone Therapy. Susan G. Komen. Accessed on May 11, 2023. https://www.komen.org/breast-cancer/risk-factor/postmenopausal-hormone-use/
6. Blakemore, E. The First Birth Control Pill Used Puerto Rican Women as Guinea Pigs. History.com. Published May 9, 2018. Updated March 11, 2019. Accessed May 11, 2023. https://www.history.com/news/birth-control-pill-history-puerto-rico-enovid
7. The Truth About Birth Control Pills and Hormones. Amen Clinics. Published November 30, 2017. Accessed May 11, 2023. https://www.amenclinics.com/blog/the-truth-about-birth-control-pills-and-hormones/

8. Chen KX, Worley S, Foster H, et al. Oral contraceptive use is associated with smaller hypothalamic and pituitary gland volumes in healthy women: A structural MRI study. PLoS One. 2021;16(4):e0249482. Published 2021 Apr 21. doi:10.1371/journal.pone.0249482
9. Skovlund CW, Mørch LS, Kessing LV, Lidegaard Ø. Association of Hormonal Contraception With Depression. JAMA Psychiatry. 2016;73(11):1154-1162. doi:10.1001/jamapsychiatry.2016.2387
10. Slap GB. Oral contraceptives and depression: impact, prevalence and cause. J Adolesc Health Care. 1981;2(1):53-64. doi:10.1016/s0197-0070(81)80087-3
11. Kenton, L. Passage to Power: Natural Menopause Revolution. Hay House, Inc. January 1, 1998.
12. Dorr B MD. In the Misdiagnosis of Menopause, What Needs to Change? AJMC.com. September 14, 2022. Accessed May 18, 2023. https://www.ajmc.com/view/contributor-in-the-misdiagnosis-of-menopause-what-needs-to-change-
13. Vance DA Dph. Premarin: the intriguing history of a controverisal drug. International Journal of Pharmaceutical Compounding. 2007;11(4):282-286.
14. Writing Group for the Women's Health Initiative Investigators. Risks and Benefits of Estrogen Plus Progestin in Healthy Postmenopausal Women: Principal Results From the Women's Health Initiative Randomized Controlled Trial. JAMA. 2002;288(3):321-333. doi:10.1001/jama.288.3.321
15. The Women's Health Initiative Steering Committee*. Effects of Conjugated Equine Estrogen in Postmenopausal Women With Hysterectomy: The Women's Health Initiative Randomized

Controlled Trial. JAMA. 2004;291(14):1701-1712. doi:10.1001/jama.291.14.1701

16. Breast Cancer in Young Women. Centers for Disease Control and Prevention. March 21, 2023. https://www.cdc.gov/cancer/breast/young_women/bringyourbrave/breast_cancer_young_women/index.htm

17. Fournier, A., Berrino, F., Riboli, E., Avenel, V., & Clavel-Chapelon, F. Breast cancer risk in relation to different types of hormone replacement therapy in the E3N-EPIC cohort. International Journal of Cancer. November 18, 2004. 114(3), 448-454. https://doi.org/10.1002/ijc.20710

18. Beral V; Million Women Study Collaborators. Breast cancer and hormone-replacement therapy in the Million Women Study [published correction appears in Lancet. 2003 Oct 4;362(9390):1160]. Lancet. 2003;362(9382):419-427. doi:10.1016/s0140-6736(03)14065-2

19. Mair KM, Gaw R, MacLean MR. Obesity, estrogens and adipose tissue dysfunction - implications for pulmonary arterial hypertension. Pulm Circ. 2020;10(3):2045894020952019. Published 2020 Sep 18. doi:10.1177/2045894020952023

20. Reeves GK, Pirie K, Beral V, Green J, Spencer E, Bull D. Cancer incidence and mortality in relation to body mass index in the Million Women Study: cohort study. BMJ. 335(7630):1134, 2007.

21. Hankinson SE, Colditz GA, Manson JE, et al. A prospective study of oral contraceptive use and risk of breast cancer. Cancer Causes Control. 8:65-72, 1997.

22. Gierisch JM, Coeytaux RR, Urrutia RP, et al. Oral contraceptive use and risk of breast, cervical, colorectal, and endometrial

cancers: a systematic review. Cancer Epidemiol Biomarkers Prev. 22(11):1931-43, 2013.

23. Combination Birth Control Pills. Mayo Clinic. January 13, 2023. https://www.mayoclinic.org/tests-procedures/combination-birth-control-pills/about/pac-20385282

24. What are the side effects of birth control pills? Brown University. 2022. Accessed May 11, 2023. https://www.brown.edu/campus-life/health/services/promotion/content/what-are-side-effects-birth-control-pills

25. Africander D, Verhoog N, Hapgood JP. Molecular mechanisms of steroid receptor-mediated actions by synthetic progestins used in HRT and contraception. Steroids. 2011;76(7):636-652. doi:10.1016/j.steroids.2011.03.001

26. Tworek, D. How to Treat Low Progesterone. January 30, 2019. Accessed May 12, 2023. https://www.bodylogicmd.com/hormones/progesterone/

27. Cable JK, Grider MH. Physiology, Progesterone. May 8, 2022. In: StatPearls. Treasure Island (FL): StatPearls Publishing; 2023 Jan-. https://www.ncbi.nlm.nih.gov/books/NBK558960/

28. Lee, JR MD., Hopkins, V. *Hormone Balance Made Simple*. 11.7.2006 edition. Balance. 2006.

29. Frisch RE. The right weight: body fat, menarche and ovulation. Baillieres Clin Obstet Gynaecol. 1990;4(3):419-439. doi:10.1016/s0950-3552(05)80302-5

30. Gonsioroski A, Mourikes VE, Flaws JA. Endocrine Disruptors in Water and Their Effects on the Reproductive System. Int J Mol Sci. 2020;21(6):1929. Published 2020 Mar 12. doi:10.3390/ijms21061929

31. Xeno-Estrogens. Georgia Strait Alliance. Accessed May 15, 2023 https://georgiastrait.org/xeno-estrogens/

32. Scialla, M. It could take centuries for EPA to test all the unregulated chemicals under a new landmark bill. PBS.org. June 22, 2016. Accessed May 15, 2023. https://www.pbs.org/newshour/science/it-could-take-centuries-for-epa-to-test-all-the-unregulated-chemicals-under-a-new-landmark-bill

33. Daley, J. Science Is Falling Woefully Behind In Testing New Chemicals. February 3, 2017. Accessed May 15, 2023. https://www.smithsonianmag.com/smart-news/science-falling-woefully-behind-testing-new-chemicals-180962027/

34. Becker, E., Lee, J. Europe Plan on Chemicals Seen as Threat to U.S. Exports. The New York Times. May 8, 2003. Accessed May 15, 2023. https://www.nytimes.com/2003/05/08/business/europe-plan-on-chemicals-seen-as-threat-to-us-exports.html

35. What are Fibroids? UCLAHealth.org. Accessed May 15, 2023. https://www.uclahealth.org/medical-services/fibroids/what-are-fibroids

36. Endometriosis. Mayoclinic.org. July 24, 2018. Accessed May 15, 2023. https://www.mayoclinic.org/diseases-conditions/endometriosis/symptoms-causes/syc-20354656

37. Fibrocycstic breast disease. Mountsinai.org. Accessed May 15, 2023. https://www.mountsinai.org/health-library/diseases-conditions/fibrocystic-breast-disease

38. Levine H, Jørgensen N, Martino-Andrade A, Mendiola J, Weksler-Derri D, Mindlis I, Pinotti R, Swan SH. Temporal trends in sperm count: a systematic review and meta-regression analysis, Human Reproduction Update, Volume 23, Issue 6,

November-December 2017, Pages 646–659, https://doi.org/10.1093/humupd/dmx022

39. Zlomislik D. Chemicals Feminizing Males, Study Suggests. Thestar.com. December 9, 2008. Accessed May 15, 2023. https://www.thestar.com/life/health_wellness/2008/12/09/chemicals_feminizing_males_study_suggests.html

40. Semenza JC, Tolbert PE, Rubin CH, Guillette LJ Jr, Jackson RJ. Reproductive toxins and alligator abnormalities at Lake Apopka, Florida. Environ Health Perspect. 1997;105(10):1030-1032. doi:10.1289/ehp.971051030

41. Guillette LJ Jr, Gross TS, Masson GR, Matter JM, Percival HF, Woodward AR. Developmental abnormalities of the gonad and abnormal sex hormone concentrations in juvenile alligators from contaminated and control lakes in Florida. Environ Health Perspect. 1994;102(8):680-688. doi:10.1289/ehp.94102680

42. Natural Sciences and Engineering Research Council. "Fish Devastated By Sex-changing Chemicals In Municipal Wastewater." ScienceDaily. February 20, 2008. Accessed May 15, 2023. www.sciencedaily.com/releases/2008/02/080216095726.htm

43. Kronzer VL, Bridges SL Jr, Davis JM 3rd. Why women have more autoimmune diseases than men: An evolutionary perspective. Evol Appl. 2020;14(3):629-633. Published 2020 Dec 1. doi:10.1111/eva.13167

44. Harding AT, Heaton NS. The Impact of Estrogens and Their Receptors on Immunity and Inflammation during Infection. Cancers (Basel). 2022;14(4):909. Published 2022 Feb 12. doi:10.3390/cancers14040909

45. Shivers KY, Amador N, Abrams L, Hunter D, Jenab S, Quiñones-Jenab V. Estrogen alters baseline and inflammatory-induced cytokine levels independent from hypothalamic-pituitary-adrenal axis activity. Cytokine. 2015;72(2):121-129. doi:10.1016/j.cyto.2015.01.007
46. Baker JM, Al-Nakkash L, Herbst-Kralovetz MM. Estrogen-gut microbiome axis: Physiological and clinical implications. Maturitas. 2017;103:45-53. doi:10.1016/j.maturitas.2017.06.025
47. Bennet J. Estrogen and the Immune System. Aria Integrative Medicine. Accessed 5/16/2023. https://www.ariaintegrative.com/2020/05/07/estrogen-and-the-immune-system
48. Hyperthyroidism vs Hypothyroidism: Here's How to Tell the Difference. Hartford Healthcare. April 29, 2021. Accessed May 16, 2023. https://hartfordhealthcare.org/about-us/news-press/news-detail?articleid=32994&publicId=395
49. Autoimmune Thyroid Diseases: What is really going on when my thyroid is not working properly. Mount Sinai Medical Center. January 11, 2016. Accessed May 16, 2023. https://www.msmc.com/autoimmune-thyroid/
50. Santin AP, Furlanetto TW. Role of estrogen in thyroid function and growth regulation. J Thyroid Res. 2011;2011:875125. doi:10.4061/2011/875125
51. Yeager MP, Pioli PA, Guyre PM. Cortisol exerts bi-phasic regulation of inflammation in humans. Dose Response. 2011;9(3):332-347. doi:10.2203/dose-response.10-013.Yeager
52. Corticosteroids. Cleveland Clinic. January 20, 2020. Accessed May 16, 2023. https://my.clevelandclinic.org/health/drugs/4812-corticosteroids

53. Hannibal KE, Bishop MD. Chronic stress, cortisol dysfunction, and pain: a psychoneuroendocrine rationale for stress management in pain rehabilitation. Phys Ther. 2014;94(12):1816-1825. doi:10.2522/ptj.20130597
54. Bianchi VE. The Anti-Inflammatory Effects of Testosterone. J Endocr Soc. 2018;3(1):91-107. Published 2018 Oct 22. doi:10.1210/js.2018-00186
55. Nasir N, Jamil B, Siddiqui S, Talat N, Khan FA, Hussain R. Mortality in Sepsis and its relationship with Gender. Pak J Med Sci. 2015;31(5):1201-1206. doi:10.12669/pjms.315.6925
56. Goldman B. In men, high testosterone can mean weakened immune response, study finds. Stanford Medicine. December 23, 2013. Accessed May 16, 2023. https://med.stanford.edu/news/all-news/2013/12/in-men-high-testosterone-can-mean-weakened-immune-response-study-finds.html
57. What is hormonal weight gain? Endocrinewellness.com. Accessed May 17, 2023. https://www.endocrinewellness.com/hormonal-weight-gain/
58. Obesity and hormones. Better Health Channel. Betterhealth.com Accessed May 17, 2023. https://www.betterhealth.vic.gov.au/health/healthyliving/obesity-and-hormones
59. Nagata C, Nagao Y, Shibuya C, Kashiki Y, Shimizu H. Fat intake is associated with serum estrogen and androgen concentrations in postmenopausal Japanese women. J Nutr. 2005;135(12):2862-2865. doi:10.1093/jn/135.12.2862
60. Jargin SV. Soy and phytoestrogens: possible side effects. Ger Med Sci. 2014;12:Doc18. Published 2014 Dec 15. doi:10.3205/000203

61. Lovallo WR, Farag NH, Vincent AS, Thomas TL, Wilson MF. Cortisol responses to mental stress, exercise, and meals following caffeine intake in men and women. Pharmacol Biochem Behav. 2006;83(3):441-447. doi:10.1016/j.pbb.2006.03.005

62. Rachdaoui N, Sarkar DK. Effects of alcohol on the endocrine system. Endocrinol Metab Clin North Am. 2013;42(3):593-615. doi:10.1016/j.ecl.2013.05.008

63. Michnovicz JJ, Bradlow HL. Altered estrogen metabolism and excretion in humans following consumption of indole-3-carbinol. Nutr Cancer. 1991;16(1):59-66. doi:10.1080/01635589109514141

64. Focus on fertility nutrition: omega-3 fatty acids. The Fertility Hub. February 3, 2021. Accessed May 17, 2023. https://thefertilityhub.com/focus-on-fertility-nutrition-omega-3-fatty-acids/

65. Gottfried S MD. The 10 Best Types of Protein for Hormone Balance. January 4, 2021. Accessed May 17, 2023. https://www.mindbodygreen.com/articles/how-protein-affects-your-hormones

66. Dyer D MD. Flaxseeds and Breast Cancer. Accessed May 17, 2023. https://www.oncologynutrition.org/erfc/healthy-nutrition-now/foods/flaxseeds-and-breast-cancer

67. Dong Y, Chen L, Gutin B, Zhu H. Total, insoluble, and soluble dietary fiber intake and insulin resistance and blood pressure in adolescents. Eur J Clin Nutr. 2019;73(8):1172-1178. doi:10.1038/s41430-018-0372-y

68. He S, Li H, Yu Z, et al. The Gut Microbiome and Sex Hormone-Related Diseases. Front Microbiol. 2021;12:711137. Published 2021 Sep 28. doi:10.3389/fmicb.2021.711137

69. Scott LA MD. Gut Health and Hormones. Leigh Ann Scott, MD. Accessed May 17, 2023. https://www.leighannscottmd.com/additional-testing/gut-health-and-hormones/

70. Khalili H. Risk of Inflammatory Bowel Disease with Oral Contraceptives and Menopausal Hormone Therapy: Current Evidence and Future Directions. Drug Saf. 2016;39(3):193-197. doi:10.1007/s40264-015-0372-y

71. Briden L. 8 Ways Magnesium Rescues Hormones. Lara Briden - The Period Revolutionary. March 30, 2014. Accessed May 17, 2023. https://www.larabriden.com/8-ways-that-magnesium-rescues-hormones/

72. Habib FK, Maddy SQ, Stitch SR. Zinc induced changes in the progesterone binding properties of the human endometrium. Acta Endocrinol (Copenh). 1980;94(1):99-106. doi:10.1530/acta.0.0940099

73. Lin MW, Wu MH. The role of vitamin D in polycystic ovary syndrome. Indian J Med Res. 2015;142(3):238-240. doi:10.4103/0971-5916.166527

74. Mumford SL, Browne RW, Schliep KC, et al. Serum Antioxidants Are Associated with Serum Reproductive Hormones and Ovulation among Healthy Women. J Nutr. 2016;146(1):98-106. doi:10.3945/jn.115.217620

75. Kim K, Mills JL, Michels KA, et al. Dietary Intakes of Vitamin B-2 (Riboflavin), Vitamin B-6, and Vitamin B-12 and Ovarian

Cycle Function among Premenopausal Women. J Acad Nutr Diet. 2020;120(5):885-892. doi:10.1016/j.jand.2019.10.013
76. Wuttke W, Jarry H, Christoffel V, Spengler B, Seidlová-Wuttke D. Chaste tree (Vitex agnus-castus)--pharmacology and clinical indications. Phytomedicine. 2003;10(4):348-357. doi:10.1078/094471103322004866
77. Herbs that Increase Progesterone: 6 astounding nutrients! DHEA Clinic. June 29, 2020. Accessed May 17, 2023. https://www.dhea.clinic/blogs/news/herbs-to-increase-progesterone
78. Mindfulness meditation: a research-proven way to reduce stress. American Psychological Association. October 30, 2019. Accessed May 17, 2023. https://www.apa.org/topics/mindfulness/meditation
79. Uvnas-Moberg K, Petersson M. Oxytocin, ein Vermittler von Antistress, Wohlbefinden, sozialer Interaktion, Wachstum und Heilung [Oxytocin, a mediator of anti-stress, well-being, social interaction, growth and healing]. Z Psychosom Med Psychother. 2005;51(1):57-80. doi:10.13109/zptm.2005.51.1.57
80. Wang SC, Zhang F, Zhu H, et al. Potential of Endogenous Oxytocin in Endocrine Treatment and Prevention of COVID-19. Front Endocrinol (Lausanne). 2022;13:799521. Published 2022 May 3. doi:10.3389/fendo.2022.799521
81. Rettori V, Canteros G, Renoso R, Gimeno M, McCann SM. Oxytocin stimulates the release of luteinizing hormone-releasing hormone from medial basal hypothalamic explants by releasing nitric oxide. Proc Natl Acad Sci U S A. 1997;94(6):2741-2744. doi:10.1073/pnas.94.6.2741

82. Scheele D, Plota J, Stoffel-Wagner B, Maier W, Hurlemann R. Hormonal contraceptives suppress oxytocin-induced brain reward responses to the partner's face. Social Cognitive and Affective Neuroscience, Volume 11, Issue 5, May 2016, Pages 767–774, https://doi.org/10.1093/scan/nsv157

83. Ennour-Idrissi K, Maunsell E, Diorio C. Effect of physical activity on sex hormones in women: a systematic review and meta-analysis of randomized controlled trials. Breast Cancer Res. 2015;17(1):139. Published 2015 Nov 5. doi:10.1186/s13058-015-0647-3

84. FDA issues final rule on safety and effectiveness of antibacterial soaps. U.S. Food & Drug Administration. September 2, 2016. Accessed May 17, 2023. https://www.fda.gov/news-events/press-announcements/fda-issues-final-rule-safety-and-effectiveness-antibacterial-soaps

85. Zhou L. Personal care product chemicals banned in Europe but still found in U.S. EWG (Environmental Working Group). October 25, 2022. Accessed May 17, 2023. https://www.ewg.org/news-insights/news/2022/10/personal-care-product-chemicals-banned-europe-still-found-us

86. Ritchie H, Roser M. Plastic Pollution. Our World In Data. Published September 2018. Updated April 2022. Accessed May 17, 2023. https://ourworldindata.org/plastic-pollution

87. Enck J, Dell J. Plastic Recycling Doesn't Work and Will Never Work. The Atlantic. May 30, 2022. https://www.theatlantic.com/ideas/archive/2022/05/single-use-plastic-chemical-recycling-disposal/661141/

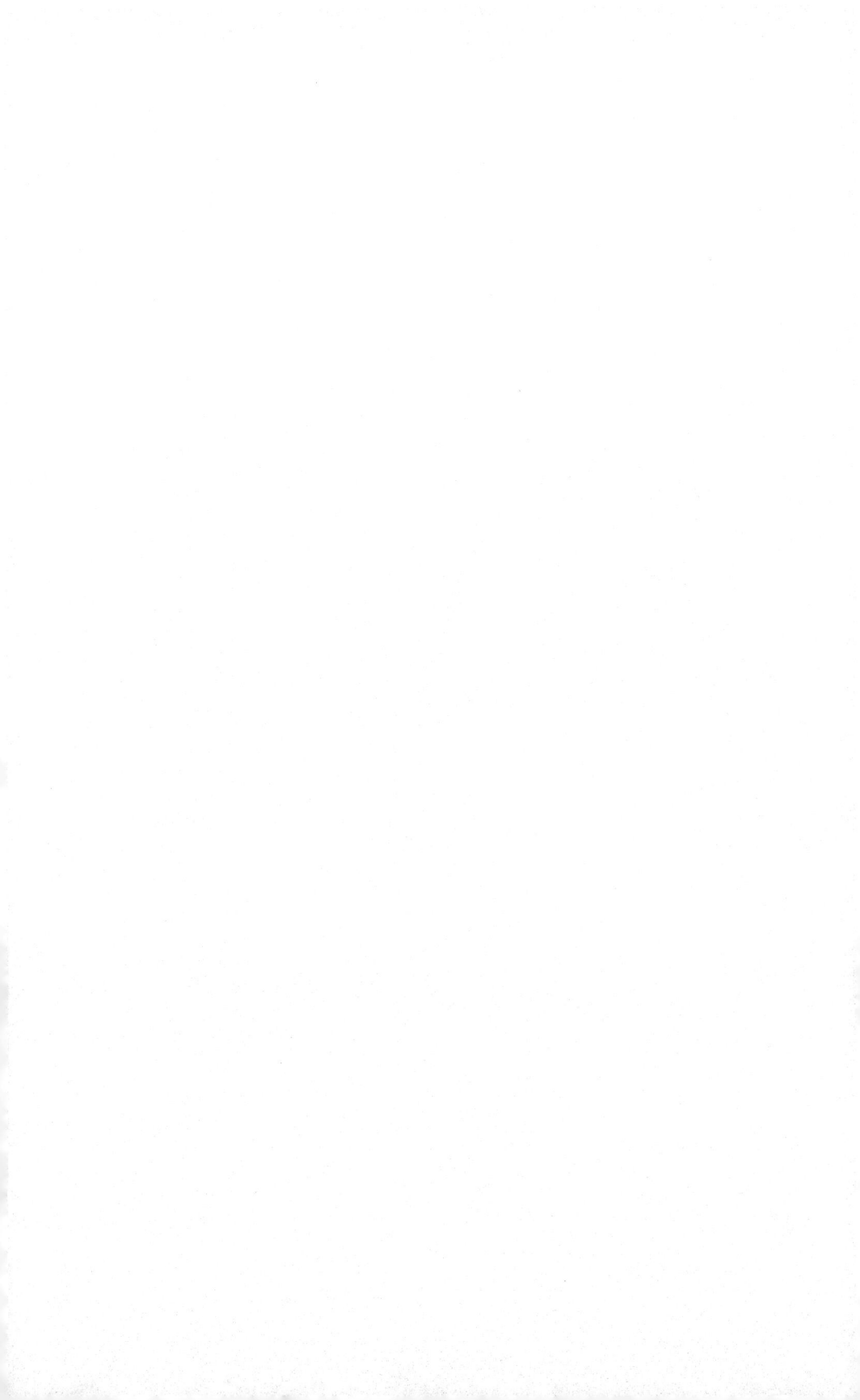

Made in the USA
Las Vegas, NV
13 August 2023